Marina

*The Qigong Way —
from body to energy to consciousness*

Max Weier

The Qigong Way –

from body
    to energy
        to consciousness

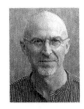 Max Weier has been studying and practicing many forms of qigong, yoga and other traditions of Eastern philosophies and mysticism, notably vipassana and Tibetan Buddhist approaches with renowned teachers and masters in the East and the West since the Eighties. From his base in his native Switzerland, he conducts retreats and workshops in Europe, Asia and Africa.

www.max-weier.com

© 2013 Max Weier

Layout, cover design, printing and publication:
BoD – Books on Demand, Germany

ISBN: 978-3-8423-8618-1

Table of contents

Acknowledgements 7

Foreword 9

The World of Qigong 11
    What is Qigong 12
    The Phenomenon of Qi 13
    The Meridians and Organs 14
    Taiji 16
    Yin and Yang 16
    Harmony 17
    Dao 17

The Way of the Body 19
    Warm-ups 20
    Standing Practice 22
    The practice of the Standing Post 23
    The Four Essential Movements 24

The Way of Energy 29
    Energy Centres 29
    Dantian 30
    Dantian Breathing 31
    The Three Dantian – The Centres of Head, Heart and Belly 32

The Harmony of Head, Heart and Belly	34
So Ham	38
Wudang Qigong	39
Daoist Alchemy – The Small Heavenly Circle	42
The Way of Consciousness	**45**
Imagination and Intention	45
Entering Stillness	46
Entering Stillness Now	47
The Work-out	**51**
Outer Preparation	51
Time and Duration	52
During and after the Session	52
Signs of Practice	53
Cleansing the Jade Body	54
Qigong and Haiku	**57**
Using Haiku Contemplation during a Qigong Session	59

Acknowledgements

I would like to thank all the people and places that have contributed in some way in helping me spread and develop my brand of qigong. My thanks go to David Francisco, Kittisaro and Thanissara, Collien Hendricks, Maren Bodenstein, Katja Abbott, Graeme Williams, Uli Hansen, to the BRC, Emoyeni, Gaia House, Casa de Espiritualidad Marratxinet and last but not least to the teachers and masters I had the good fortune to learn from.

Foreword

This work attempts to present in a concise form the basic principles of qigong and the theory behind it. Illustrated with photos and drawings and underpinned with short instructions it can serve as an introduction into the practice of qigong or as a manual to inspire and refine one's own practice.

The exercises presented here have been taken from or inspired by different schools, styles or practices within the vast qigong tradition, such as Daoyin Yangsheng Gong, Wudang Qigong, Taoist Yoga and others.

Today qigong, like most modern yoga styles, focuses almost exclusively on health, leaving out wider aspects of the practice. Hence, in addition to the physical and energetic exercises with their remarkably calming, invigorating and healing benefits, some meditational practices originating in the shamanist, Daoist and Buddhist traditions are also described and incorporated here. Furthermore, the ultimate goal of qigong: returning to one's Original Nature is briefly touched upon. Eventually qigong can free us from our ego-centred world and open us to the deeper dimensions of who we are.

This book hopes to offer a fresh and more integrated approach to the ancient art of qigong.

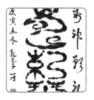

The World of Qigong

Often qigong is compared to a great river that is fed by four streams:

- » Shamanism
- » Spirituality (Daoism and Buddhism)
- » Medicine
- » The Martial Arts

The first qigong practices, the first conscious energy-work, was done by shamans. In pre-historic North-East Asia shamans used to imitate animal movements in slow motion during their ritual dances. They discovered that through these emulations they could increase their life-force and, in turn, utilize the amplified internal energy for healing and exorcism.

Later Daoist hermits adapted the archaic shamanist movements, developed new exercises and practices and imbued them with Daoist concepts. After Indian Buddhism was established in China a number of monks resorted to these ancient exercises to keep healthy and as an aid for their long meditation retreats.

From its early beginnings qigong practice entered the arena of healing and over the centuries it became an important part of Chinese medicine as a preventative and self-healing method.

Fighters and folk who had been forced to defend themselves against enemies and bandits have been inspired by qigong practices, converting them into martial arts techniques and creating new exercises.

There has always been, all along the history of qigong, a cross-pollination with the other disciplines.

Today a fifth tributary is contributing to the Great River of qigong: the adaptation, modification and enrichment of this age-old art through its contact with modern Western culture. Confronted with an abundance of styles and brands of qigong, with yoga, different forms of meditation and spiritual teachings, with psychotherapy and all kinds of bodywork, qigong is developing its own integral expressions and flavour in the Western world.

What is Qigong

> *Qigong is the cultivation of one's life-force.*
> *It is the holistic experience of body, energy, heart and mind.*

Our organism is a unity in which everything is physically and energetically interconnected. Hence the quality and mobility of our life-force impacts on how we feel physically, emotionally and mentally. If there is a free and even flow of qi through the system we feel at ease and in balance. If the internal energy is blocked i.e. due to emotional stress we are out of sync.

The practices of qigong help to dissolve blockages and to restore the natural flow of the life-force. At the same time they affect the blood and the lymphatic system and strengthen the bone marrow and the inner organs. Frequently, suppressed emotions that are stored deep in our tissue get released. Through qigong exercises the body relaxes, tensions ease and the mind can become tranquil.

Most qigong movements are done in a slow, soft and concentrated way, often coordinated with deep breathing. Slow movements have the capacity to access and powerfully increase one's internal energy. At the same time they switch the nervous system from the stressful 'fight or flight' response to the energy restoring 'rest and digest' mode. In addition, slow-motion helps modern humans to slow down internally and become more conscious of themselves and the environment.

In the same way that each organism is a unity, it is also part of the greater web of life intimately linked to the Ten Thousand Things, to the universe.

> *Qigong is the cultivation of a consciousness realising that we are part of life, deeply connected to everything.*

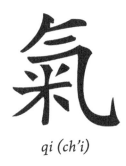

qi (ch'i)

The Phenomenon of Qi

The phenomenon of *qi* – life-force, or energy flow – can be found in many cultures. In the Indian Vedas it is called *prana*, the Tibetan Buddhists call it *lung*. *Qi* is the formative force behind all manifestation.

> *Qi is the basis and support of all life.*

> *Qi is the interface between matter and its source.*

We are all born with a certain amount of *qi*. Found in all our organs, bones, joints and subtle energy-centres it is stored to a great part in the kidneys. Our innate stamina and our constitution largely depend on the level and quality of our kidney *qi*.

There are also external sources of *qi* we depend on. Like the *qi* we extract from the air we breathe, we absorb *qi* from the liquids we drink and form the food we eat. The purer the air and the water, the less processed the food, the higher the quality of their *qi*.

And finally there is the *qi* produced through the harmonious movements of the body-mind through walking and exercise which we assimilate.

The Meridians and Organs

The *qi* flows through our body in a sophisticated network of channels, the meridians, providing our whole organism with life-energy. Under ideal conditions the *qi* moves freely in its pathways. If the flow is blocked the consequences for body and mind are, in one way or another, disharmonious.

The main meridians are named after the five organs: lungs, kidneys, liver, heart and spleen. Every organ possesses a counterpart, is responsible for a whole range of different functions; has a *yin* and *yang* side; and has specific qualities associated with it. The term 'organ circuit' comprises the (double-)organ, its meridians and energy-points and certain functions and characteristics like emotions etc.

The lungs, for instance, are considered the *yin* part of the lung organ circuit, and the large intestines are the *yang* part. The element pertaining to the lungs is air. The positive emotional quality is seen as courage and the negative as sadness. The season associated with the lung is autumn and the colour is white. Furthermore every organ is linked to a sense organ, a climate, a tissue, a liquid emitted and a taste.

The elements should not be considered material substances but forces that give direction to the natural phenomena.

Organ yin yang	Element Force	Season Climate	Colour	Sense org	Emotion
Lungs Large intestines	Metal contracting	Autumn dry	white	nose	+ courage - sorrow
Kidneys Bladder	Water descending	Winter cold	blue	ear	+ rootedness - fear
Liver Gallbladder	Wood expanding	Spring windy	green	eyes	+ generosity - anger
Heart Small Intestines	Fire ascending	Summer hot	red	tongue	+ love - hate
Spleen Stomach	Earth stabilising	Indian Summer damp	yellow	mouth	+ trust - worry

Taiji

Mostly, dynamic practices in qigong consist of a number of particular movements where every movement is individually repeated various times. If the different movements flow one into the other and if the isolated gesture can be applied within a martial arts context the exercise becomes taiji. Thus taiji is nothing but qigong principles converted into a soft martial art and its results – the harmonisation of body and mind, relaxation, alertness and a sense of groundedness – are the same as in qigong. Not seldom today taiji is deliberately carried without its martial spirit purely as an albeit sophisticated, qigong exercise.

Yin and Yang

Qigong is based on a holistic worldview and of its most popular principles is the concept of *yin* and *yang*. The philosophy behind this is that the manifest world has its origins in the interplay between the two polar forces of *yin* and *yang*. It is the dynamic interaction between the two poles that creates the *qi* and makes it flow. Polarity applies to every process and phenomenon in the universe: earth and space, water and fire, night and day, woman and man, cold and hot, left and right, empty and full, below and above etc. Through qigong movements we express and experience the alternation of *yin* and *yang* continuously: in lifting and sinking, stretching and bending, opening and closing, tensing and relaxing. By alternating and balancing the two polar forces we balance our own body-mind.

yin-yang

> *To balance yin and yang is a key principle in qigong.*

Harmony

Qigong seeks harmony and balance within the micro-cosmos of the body-mind and harmony between the body-mind and the macro-cosmos of manifestation. To be in harmony with oneself and with the universe is a pivotal point in the Daoist spiritual view. In its constant change and movement, life always strives towards balance.

> *In qigong we facilitate life's inherent swing towards harmony.*

Dao

Dao is the primordial ground. It is the cause of everything that is. It is the absolute principle. The concept of the Dao can't be understood by the mind. It can only be realised through mystical insight. The word Dao also signifies 'the way things are and unfold in the universe'. Furthermore the word Dao simply means 'the way', the path one treads in order to meet the Source.

zen circle

> *Dao is the source of the Ten Thousand Things and at the same time it pervades all manifestation.*

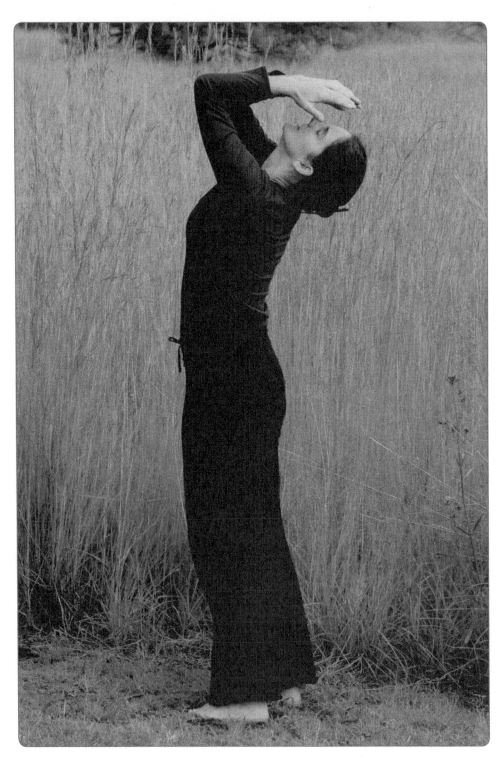

Qi feeds the Spirit

The Way of the Body

Qigong practice should always start with making conscious contact with one's body. Too many people today are out of touch with their bodies. It is as if they live in cocoon of thoughts away from their physical existence. This disturbed relationship with one's own body manifests in society's loss of connection to the larger body of the earth, resulting in the dire destruction of our planet's ecological system.

Many of us don't realise how tense our bodies have become and how paralysed our *qi* is. The stressful situations of modern life, in combination with the crowdedness of big cities and the level of fear and aggression we are exposed to, create the ideal conditions for our bodies to tighten into neuro-muscular tensions and for the *qi* to dam up.

> There is a small barren cell with some derelict wooden benches along the grey walls. A bright, cold neon-light gleams from the ceiling. Sixteen inmates of a high security prison in Johannesburg, South Africa have come together here to practice qigong exercises and meditation for one morning.
>
> The prisoners in front of me wear their orange prison uniforms covered all over with words in black letters like big black round stamps saying 'prisoner'. They are tensed-up. They spend all day in hopelessly overcrowded cells with forty to fifty other inmates. We start practicing. I notice sketchy movements, uncoordinated as if retarded by some invisible force. The bodies are stiff, the *qi* is paralysed. After an hour or so of exercises the prisoner's bodies begin to loosen up and their *qi* starts to move. There is a palpable shift of energy now in the dingy room. When the inmates sit down on the wooden benches and close their eyes for moments of just sitting still, I can see the relaxation in their faces and bodies. I can feel that life has returned to them again.

Warm-ups

Warm-ups are exercises that open the body, connecting its different parts and prepare it for the actual qigong practice.

A selection of warm-ups

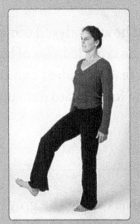 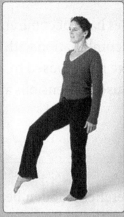 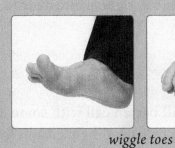 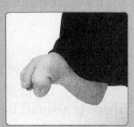

rotate ankle — *wiggle toes*

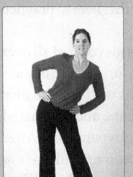 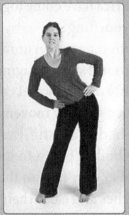 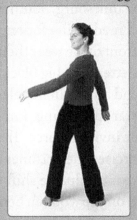 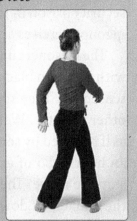

circle hips — *swing arms around*

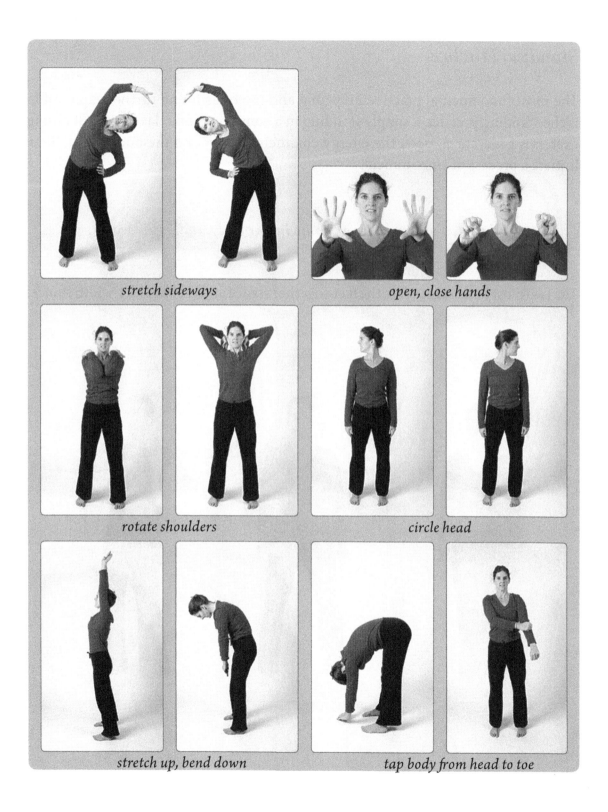

Standing Practice

The most fundamental practice in qigong and the basis for all further exploration is the standing practice – simply standing in a conscious and relaxed way. Standing exercises generate *qi*, open the energy channels and ground the body-mind. They initiate a process of embodiment.

> *Being well rooted we are more at home in our body and in the world.*

The two most basic stances are the feet-together stance and the shoulder-width stance.

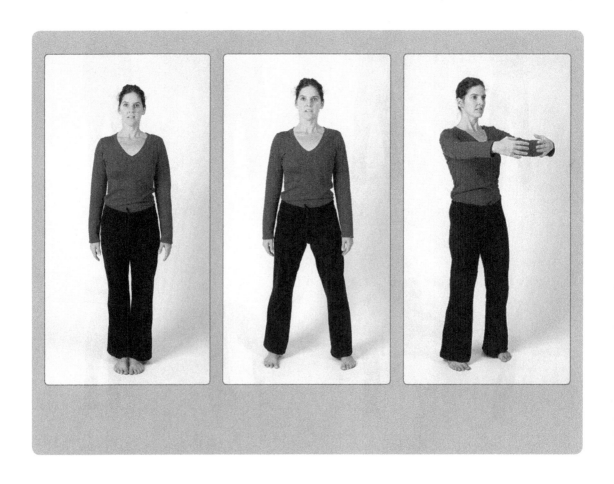

The practice of the Standing Post

- » Assume the shoulder-width stance, bending knees
- » The shoulders are relaxed, the tailbone is rooted into the ground
- » Let go in the lumbar region. Imagine leaning against a wall
- » The head is held as though suspended from a thread attached to the crown of the head like a puppet on a string
- » Think of the upper part of the body as light, the lower part as firm. The dividing line between above and below is at the level of the navel. The lower part is influenced by the earth force, the upper part by the heavens

Above light – Below firm

- » Raise arms until hands are in front of the chest, elbows bent, hands facing the body
- » Imagine holding a large inflatable beach ball cradled in your arms and pressed against the upper torso. Leave space under your armpits
- » Fingers are soft, rounded and spread

Smile at the beginning of your standing session. Smiling releases the hormone serotonin which relaxes the muscles. If you don't want to or if you can't smile, imagine water flowing down your body. This has a similar effect on the organism as smiling.

Our system absorbs the *qi* in around us through the whole body, but especially through specific energy-points on the meridians – like the top of the head, the perineum, the sacrum, the point opposite the navel and through areas like the palms of the hands and the soles of the feet.

- » Breathe with your toes, fingers and your hair, your scalp. Breathe with your whole skin. Breathe into your bones. Imagine inhaling golden-white light and exhaling black smoke
- » Feel how your feet touch the ground. Feel your whole body. Be present in every cell of your body.

> *Embodiment starts when the body-mind becomes increasingly conscious.*

The Four Essential Movements

The Four Essential Movements originate in the Baduanjin Qigong style. They engage the body in four different ways:

- » pushing
- » stretching
- » bending
- » twisting

These exercises work on the tendons, the joints and the muscles. They unblock the meridians and energy-centres, stimulate the *qi* and help it circulate. They are the ideal preparation for the more subtle and internal forms of qigong.

The Four Essential Movements:

Two Hands Hold up the Heavens

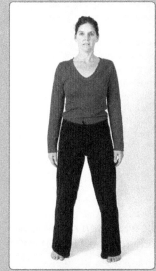

start in shoulder width stance

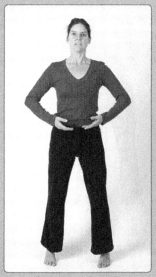

with palms facing up move hands upwards while rising onto toes

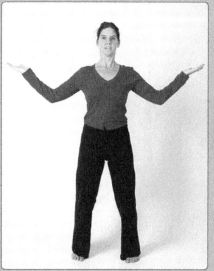

at ribcage height move hands out to the sides and come back onto heels again

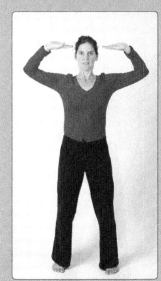

keep palms facing up and rotate hands so fingers point to temples

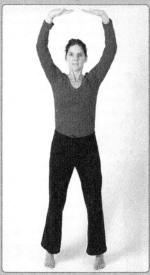

push up with both hands while rising up onto toes

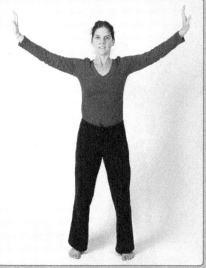

release arms out sideways and down to the thighs to starting position

The Way of the Body

Turn between Heaven and Earth

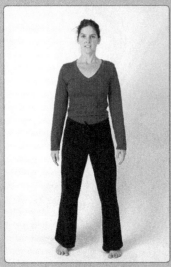

start in shoulder width stance

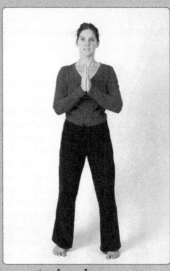

raise hands to prayer position at chest

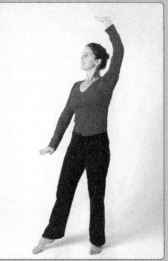

take weight on right leg as body turns on ball of left foot towards the left. at the same time extend right arm upwards palm facing sky while left arm drops down palm facing earth. head turns to the left

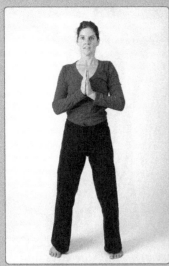

return to prayer position and make movement to the right

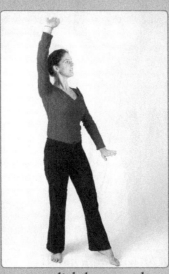

gaze slightly upwards

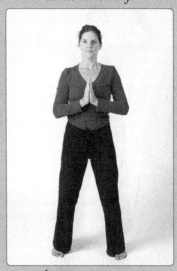

end at prayer position

Raise and Bend and Make the Back Strong

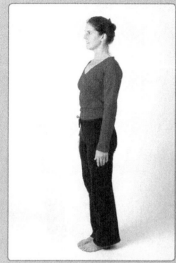

feet together, arms relaxed at the sides

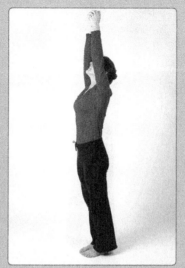

turn palms out and raise arms up the sides of the body. interlace fingers above head and look at sky

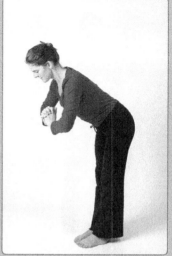

drop elbows down and start to bend forwards as interlaced hands move down the centre line of the body

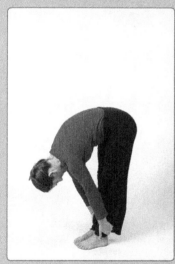

at maximum forward bend release hands

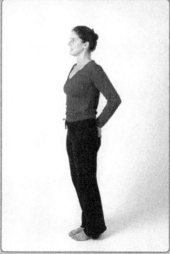

come upright with hands wiping up the back of the legs, buttocks and kidneys

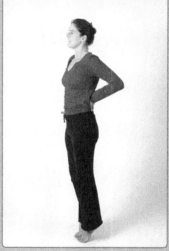

when hands wipe over kidneys rise up onto toes. when hands wipe down over kidneys and buttocks come back onto heels

The Way of the Body

Touch Moon and Earth Together

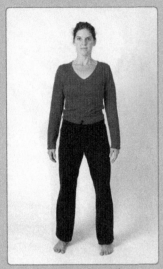

start in shoulder width stance

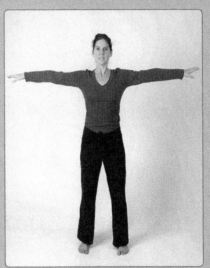

lift arms out sideways to shoulder height

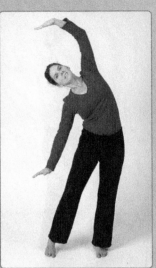

take weight on right leg while lifting left heel and start bending upper body to left. keep shoulders facing straight forwards

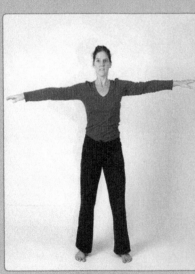

move back to position of arms held out sideways

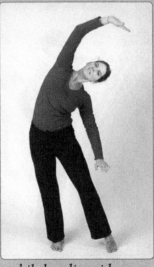

while bending sideways the upper arm curves over to the other side. palms are facing the moon respectively the earth

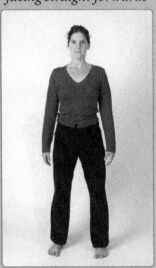

end in the starting position

The Way of Energy

The main purpose of qigong is to build up and move the *qi* in our system. Through the increase and circulation of *qi* subtle knots in the meridians and energy-centres dissolve allowing a free flow of the life-force.

Normally it doesn't take a long time to feel the surge of the internal energy in the system. First we might feel the *qi* as a current of energy in a particular part of our body. It could be the hands or the chest or any other area. When the flow of the life-force has become more powerful and unobstructed we realise that our physical body is actually one mass of vibration, a scintillating field of energy. In the past our body felt heavy, resisting and dense. Now it is light, porous and like expanded in space.

Energy Centres

Like the chakras of the Indian tantric systems, energy-centres also play an important part in many qigong practices. The locations of most of the main subtle centres are congruent with the well-known Indian chakra map. However, there are some peculiarities in the qigong tradition. Like the energy-field of the perineum, the point opposite the navel, the point at the lower back of the head and above all the centre in the lower belly. The core of the lower belly is of particular importance. It is called the *dantian*.

Dantian

The *dantian* lies at the root of qigong practice and its discovery originates in prehistoric Eastern shamanism. The centre in the lower belly is the major generator and storage place for *qi* in our energy system. At the same time the *dantian* is also the gravity-centre of our physical body.

The sphere of the *dantian* is roughly the size of a grapefruit and its core is located more or less three finger-width below the navel. To concentrate on any point within the field of the *dantian* activates its energy. The navel, which is part of the *dantian*-sphere, is an excellent anchor point to get in touch with the *qi*-power in the lower belly.

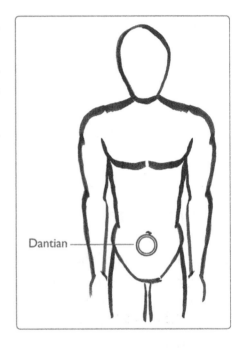

*Resting in the **dantian** we feel more powerful and grounded.*

In order to have a potent *dantian* we have to develop a strong pelvic floor. Tightening the perineum and the anus helps to strengthen the pelvic floor and simultaneously facilitates the generation of *qi*. Another way to develop and increase *dantian* power is to use our breathing.

Dantian Breathing

The two most common breathing techniques in qigong are <u>normal</u> and <u>reverse</u> breathing.

In <u>normal breathing</u> our lower belly rises on the in-breath and falls on the out-breath. Extending the inhalation and the expansion of the lower abdomen activates the *dantian*.

In <u>reverse breathing</u> we contract the lower belly while we inhale, and expand it while we exhale. This is a very potent *dantian* fuelling exercise.

> *Before and after qigong practice always root yourself in the belly.*

In the Japanese Zen Buddhist tradition the energy centre of the *dantian* is called *hara*. Its cultivation plays an essential part in Zen meditation as well as in the martial arts.

> *I remember when I was in my twenties and embarking on Zen meditation, my Japanese master taught us to keep our awareness in the lower belly at all times, to live totally from the hara like the samurai did. He said that being firmly rooted in the belly would bestow us with a sense of security, centredness, presence and power. I tried the hara exercise every now and then. When I was walking down a busy street in a city I frequently used to focus on my lower belly... and lo and behold most of the times when I was doing this practice people where automatically moving away from me, yielding their space! I could not have had a more graphic example of hara-power.*

The Three Dantian – The Centres of Head, Heart and Belly

Although there are two other vital energy-centres labelled *dantian*, it's usually the energy-field in the lower belly which is referred to by that term. It is the <u>lower</u> *dantian* that one predominantly works with in qigong, the foundation on which practice of the other two *dantian*, the <u>middle</u> and the <u>higher</u>, rests. These are located in the middle of the chest and the head.

The locations of the three *dantian* can differ from school to school.

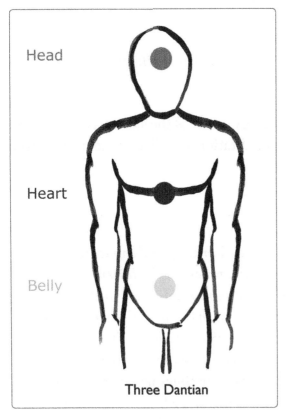

Three Dantian

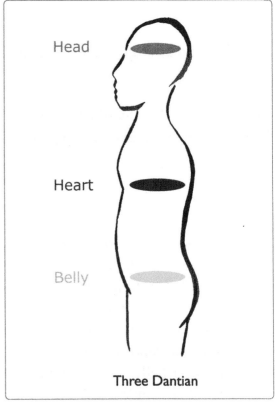

Three Dantian

Belly	Heart	Head
lower	middle	higher
Connecting to the ground Physical embodiment	Connecting to the manifestation Emotional embodiment	Connecting to the heavens Cognitive embodiment
Source of energy	Source of love and compassion	Source of wisdom and insight
pre-personal	personal	impersonal

» It is the belly centre from where we connect to the ground and from where we embody ourselves physically.
» It is the heart centre from where we connect to our emotions and from where we relate to the world.
» It is the head centre from where we connect to our mind and from where we think and discern.

The Harmony of Head, Heart and Belly

The three *dantian* can be seen as gateways into specific enlightened aspects of our body-mind organism.

In the qigong practice 'The Harmony of the Three Dantian' we awaken and align the centres of head, heart and belly. In the process of cultivation, a purification of the three energy-fields and its disharmonious qualities takes place. Physical disembodiment, destructive emotions and mental afflictions get transformed into the harmonious expressions of the three *dantian*. Through the cultivation and integration of the belly, heart and head centres we are able to inhabit life fully, freely and fluidly.

> *To inhabit life fully: **physically, emotionally, mentally**.*

palms out

Fill the Belly with Qi

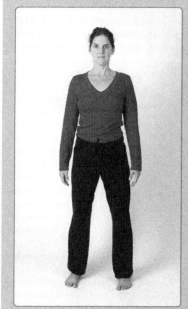

start in shoulder width stance, knees slightly bent

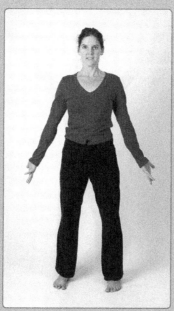

turn palms out

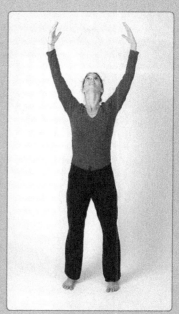

move arms sideways above head

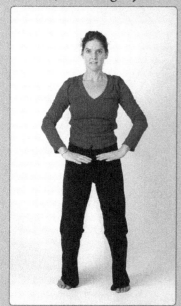

with palms facing earth draw qi down into lower belly

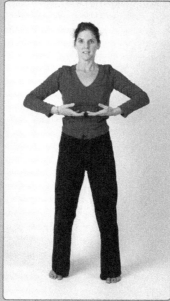

turn palms up, raise hands to base of sternum

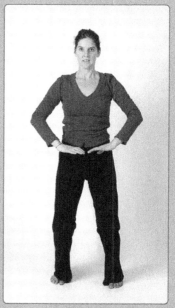

turn palms down, sink into knees and push down to lower belly

hands back to back

Fill the Heart with Qi

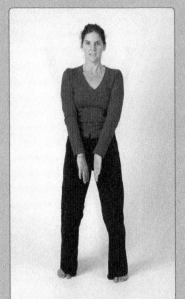
back of hands are facing each other

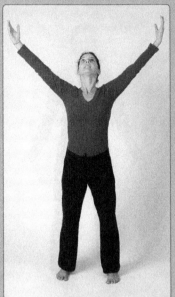
raise arms into a wide V, channel heavenly qi into heart centre

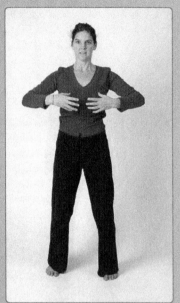
hands move to heart centre, fingertips facing each other

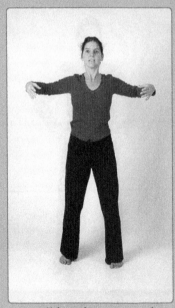
pull hands apart and open chest wide

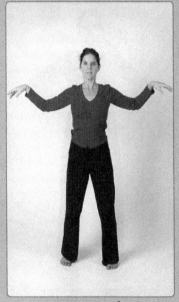
turn wrists so fingers point down

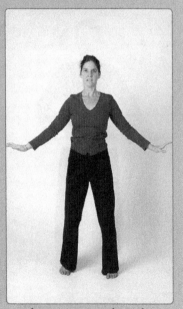
drop arms to the sides

Max Weier • The Qigong Way - from body to energy to consciousness

scooping hands

Fill the Crown with Qi

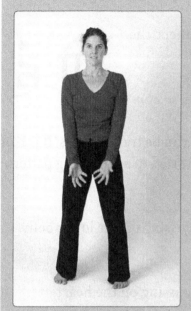

turn both palms forward

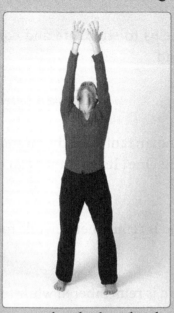

scoop hands above head

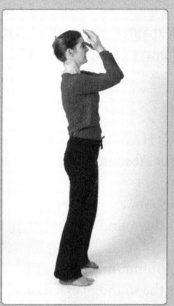

lower elbows and place palms in front of forehead

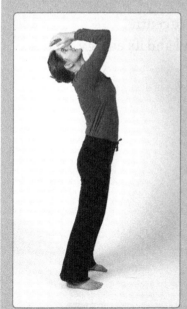

hold position of hands, tilt head back

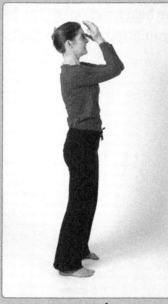

return to central position, palms facing forehead

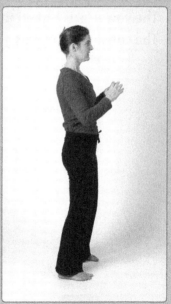

release hands and drop, palms facing downwards

The Way of Energy

So Ham

A mantra meditation that helps to stimulate and connect the centres of belly, heart and head

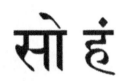

Sanskrit letters 'so ham'

SO HAM is a mantra in the Indian tantric tradition and can be translated as 'It is I' or 'the Absolute Reality and I are One'. Its utterance can be tied to a breathing pattern:

Soooo...
is the sound of inhalation, and is remembered while focussing on the lower belly.

Hummmm...
is the sound of exhalation, and is remembered while focussing on the heart.

The vowel 'o' is associated with the belly area and automatically energizes the belly and its corresponding energy-field.
    The vowel 'a' is linked to the heart and opens the heart-centre.
    The consonant 'm' has a stimulating effect on the head and its energy centres.

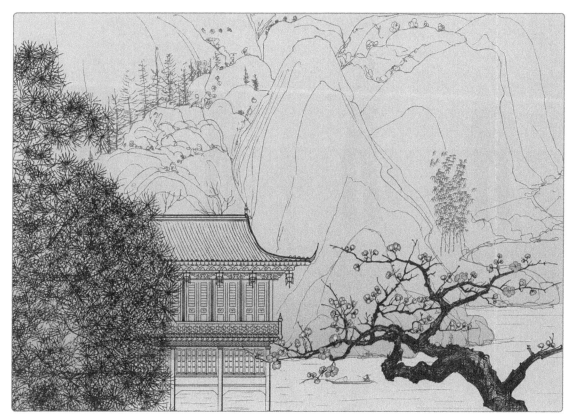
Chinese painting

Wudang Qigong

Wudang Qigong is an umbrella term for numerous styles of qigong emerging from the Daoist monasteries and hermitages on Wudang mountain.

The following Wudang Qigong exercises don't involve strenuous bodily movements. They gently, easily and powerfully generate *qi* and deeply calm the mind. These practices can also be done in any sitting position (on a chair or cross-legged on the floor).

Raise and Sweep the Qi:

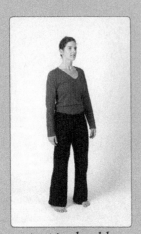
start in shoulder width stance

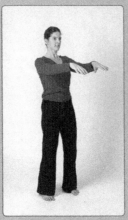
palms facing the earth, arms float up in front of body to shoulder height

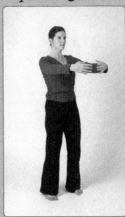
turn palms to face chest

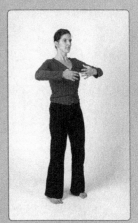
move hands in towards chest and sweep palms down in front of the body

Circle at the Horizon:

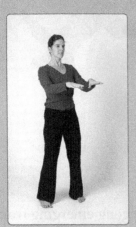
raise both hands to belly level, palms facing the earth

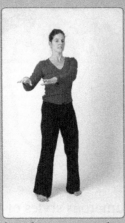
hands move together from left to right, drawing a circle

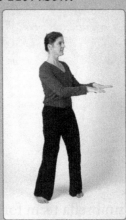
circle a few times to the left, then start circling to the right

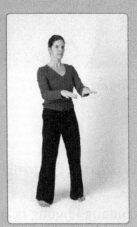
drop hands in front of you

Rising like Mist - Falling like Snow

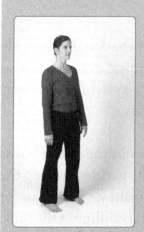 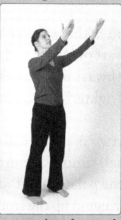 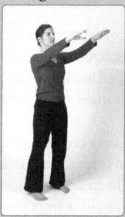 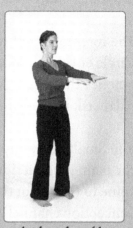

| start in shoulder width stance | turn palms forwards and lightly raise arms upwards to the sky | turn palms down | let hands softly float down |

Open and Close Hands - Gather the Qi

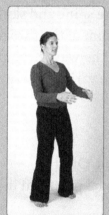 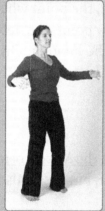 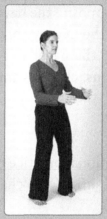 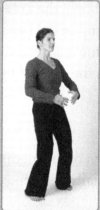 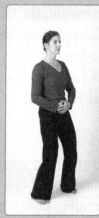

| start in shoulder width stance. palms face each other at level of belly. relax shoulders and keep a feeling of space between arms and body | expand hands outward to the sides | bring hands back in towards each other. keep on expanding and contracting hands. sense the qi-field developing between palms | condense the qi-field in front of lower belly. gradually shift qi-field into dantian | place one hand on dantian and other hand on top. breathe into hands |

The Way of Energy

Daoist Alchemy – The Small Heavenly Circle

The foremost method of qigong meditation is the practice of the Small Heavenly Circle or the Microcosmic Orbit. It is the heart of Daoist alchemical exercise. In this practice the *qi* gets guided along certain pathways of the energy-system and thereby balanced, refined and transformed into a 'brighter' consciousness.

The Small Heavenly Circle consists of the two main meridians in the subtle body: the main *yang*-meridian (or governor channel) running from the perineum along the spine to the top of the head and ending at the palate; and the main *yin*-meridian (or conception channel) stretching from the perineum up the frontal midline of the torso to the tip of the tongue. These two meridians are the channels that grow first in the energy-body of an embryo.

In the Microcosmic Orbit meditation the *qi*, sometimes visualised as a pearl of light, is taken along the two pathways and through their respective energy-centres: the perineum, the tailbone, the area opposite the navel, the point where spine and skull join together, the top of the head, the mid-eye brow point, the bottom of the throat, the heart centre, the solar plexus, the navel and the *dantian*. On the way through the two meridians the *qi* pearl opens, cleanses and balances out the various energy-centres.

<u>A simplified version of the meditational practice of the Microcosmic Orbit</u>
The exercise is usually performed sitting on a chair, but it can also be practiced in a standing position.

- » We become aware of the perineum and contract its muscles a few times.
- » With a long inhalation we take our breath from the perineum up the back along the centre line of the body to the crown of the head.
- » With the exhalation we let the breath drop down the front centre line of the body to the perineum making a full circle or orbit.
- » While we move our attention and breath along the circuit our tongue is gently placed into the roof of the mouth in order to connect the *yang* and *yin* channels.

» We repeat this exercise as many times as feels suitable.
» We let the last round finish at the *dantian* where we collect the *qi* by placing our awareness into the *dantian* and by circling our hands on the lower belly in both directions.

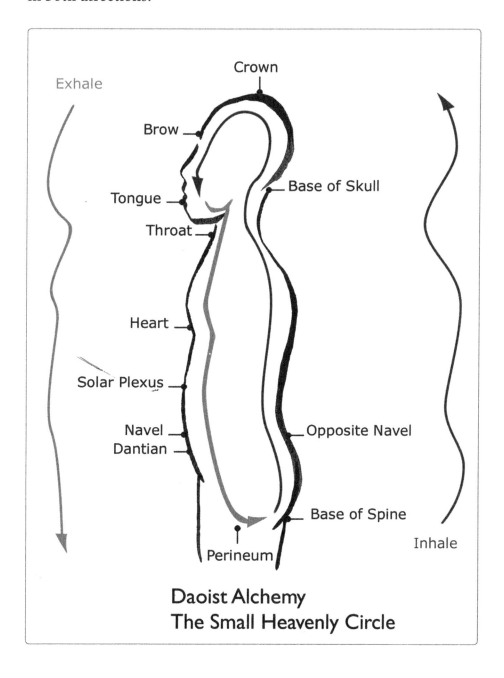

Daoist Alchemy
The Small Heavenly Circle

The Way of Consciousness

Snow covers the earth and sky,
Everything is new.
My body is concealed inside a silver world.
Suddenly I enter a treasury of light.
A place forever free of any trace of dust.
Han Shan Dejing, Buddhist monk (1546-1623), China

Sometimes as physical tensions dissolve and the *qi* gets unblocked through qigong practice, repressed emotions arise and dissolve as well. On the other hand thoughts and emotions trigger off responses in our physiology. If we think of something pleasant or unpleasant, imagine situations that had been delightful or irritating our body and its energy will react accordingly and either open and relax or close and contract.

Imagine intensely fire and you will feel warmer, ice and you will experience a breeze of cold.

Imagination and Intention

Imagination, the strategic use of inner images, is a powerful tool in qigong to intensify the effect of the practice.

The *qi* always follows the movement of our mind. It is our intention that guides the *qi*. Wherever we put our awareness the *qi* will automatically manifest.

> *Where our mind goes the qi follows.*

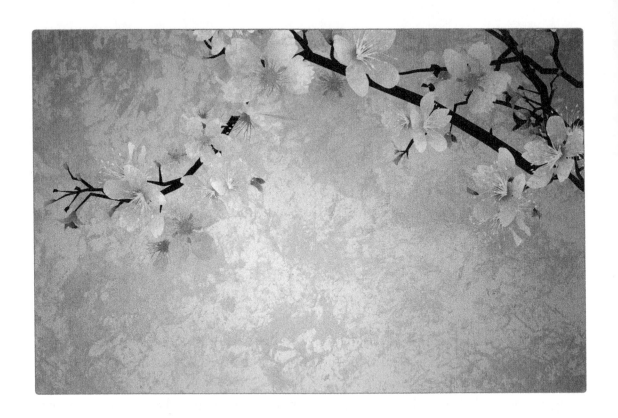

Entering Stillness

The ultimate aim of qigong is called 'Entering Stillness' (chin. *ru ching*).

The generation of *qi*
Its free and even flow in the system
The balancing of body and mind

all of it leads to and culminates in discovering the Stillness within ourselves and its integration into our daily lives.

A body-mind that has cultivated collectedness, clarity and balance is more likely to access its inherent Stillness and assimilate it than an organism that is contracted and agitated.

Finally 'Entering Stillness' means to realize our True Nature. It means to enter and rest in our impersonal Beingness.

Stillness is the background from which our life and the world continuously emerge:

- the sensations of the physical body
- the pulsation of *qi*
- the hearing, smelling and tasting
- the emotions and thoughts

Stillness is like the outer silence within which the sounds arise and pass away. Being aware of our own Stillness leads us to the centre of everything, to the Dao. Stillness and the Dao are one.

Entering Stillness Now

- Relax
- Feel your entire body from head to toes
- Listen
- Listen to everything around you
- Listen with your skin
- Listen into space
- Let the rigid edges of your body-mind dissolve
- Relax
- Open your awareness
- Include all that arises: sounds, sensations, emotions, thoughts
- Leave everything just as it is
- Witness
- Relax
- Witness
- Be
- Now

Be empty – be still.
Watch everything just come and go.
Emerging from the Source, returning to the Source.
This is the Way of the Dao.
Lao Zhi, Dao de Jing, verse 16

> *I am more than my story. I am the conscious Stillness in which my life happens.*

> *I am embodied Presence*

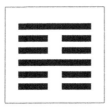

KEEPING STILL
Hexagram 52 in the Yi Jing (I Ging)

> *from the Yi Jing (I Ging)*
> *Hexagram 52: Keeping Still*
>
> *The Judgement*
>
> *Keeping one's back still*
> *So that restlessness dissolves;*
> *Then, beyond the tumult,*
> *One perceives the great laws.*
>
> When one has become calm one can turn to the outside world again. No longer does one see in it the struggle and tumult of individual beings. One has the true internal peace necessary for understanding the great laws of the universe and for acting in harmony with them. He who acts from this deep level of stillness makes no mistakes. When movement and rest accord with the time their course becomes bright and clear.

Grounded in Stillness we 'act without doing' (chin. *wu wei*). Our actions come from a deeper source in us. Untainted by a 'me' whatever we do is in harmony with the flow of events.
"Deeds are done, events happen – but there is no doer thereof" (the Buddha).

The Way of Consciousness

Morning Chi x 2

Gathering
Wave Breath
4 essential movements Flow x 4
Storing = Wood position in between
Rising like mist, Falling like Snow
Filling the belly with Chi
Abdominal Massage
Gathering

The Work-out

> *Learning and practicing qigong consists of three phases:*
> 1. *Acquiring the particular exercise with its sequence (effort).*
> 2. *Internalising it so that it becomes automated (non-tension bound effort).*
> 3. *Being aware of the effect on the body-mind (relaxed presence).*

Outer Preparation

The ideal place for practice is outside in a natural environment where *qi* is most abundant. But it is not advised to exercise in the open under abnormal meteorological conditions like in a gale, or in extreme heat or cold. Neither should one practice, even inside, during a thunderstorm. Aberrant environmental energies could enter into circulation in the human energy-system and cause disturbances and imbalances.

Wear loose fitting clothes and practice either barefoot or with flat shoes.

Never exercise on a full stomach. The last meal should have been reasonably well digested.

Drink a glass of water or tea before embarking on the practice to stimulate the *qi* in the kidneys.

Time and Duration

The best time for qigong is just before sunrise when the *qi* in the atmosphere is purest. The second best time is around sunset.

Exercising for 20 to 30 minutes is enough but try to practice on a daily basis. Continuity is the key to success.

During and after the Session

If you wish to, play some inspiring music that you find congruent with your practice. Sounds have an enormous influence on our organism and emotions. The 'right' kind of music is capable of opening our body-mind and to harmonise the *qi*-flow.

Always end the session by collecting the *qi* in the *dantian*. Anchor the vital energy in your lower belly where it will remain for the rest of the day.

If you have to interrupt your session abruptly due to an unexpected intrusion from the outside go back to the practice after attending to the matter and finish in the formal way.

Don't throw yourself into activity right after exercising. Have a quiet transition period: meditate, lie down, or have something to drink or just sit leisurely for a few minutes. Change consciously from the active *yang*-phase of the practice to the *yin*-phase, the period of stillness and rest – the time when the *qi* generated integrates with the body-mind.

If you do dynamic and more meditative exercises in the same session, start with the dynamic ones first. Move from the more physical to the more subtle, and finally from movement to stillness.

Signs of Practice

The signs of working with *qi* are manifold.

Besides a feeling of balance and tranquillity, hot, cold or tingling sensations in the hands and feet are very common.

Warm sweat, insomnia, tiredness, dizziness, headache, trembling and sexual stimulation can be side effects of the practice.

Sometimes the surge of *qi*-power causes deep internal shifting by activating and releasing the repressed emotions in our physical tissue.

Normally the problems and discomfort disappear once our system has got used to the higher intake of *qi*-energy and once the blockages have been dissolved and the numb areas in our body have become alive again.

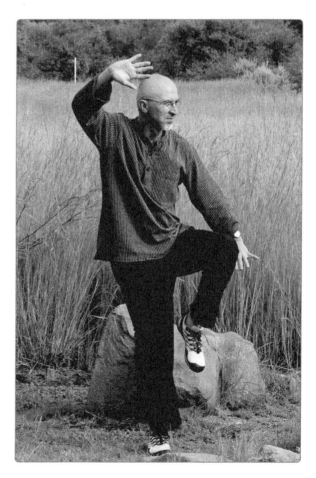

receiving the Heaven's qi

The Work-out

Cleansing the Jade Body

This qigong exercise stimulates the three *dantian* and the flow of *qi* across the whole body.

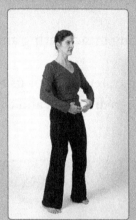
start in shoulder width stance, palms facing lower belly

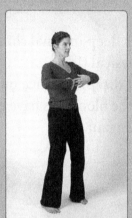
move hands up to chest, fingers pointing towards the heart

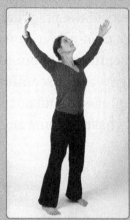
open arms into a V-position, receiving heavenly qi into the heart

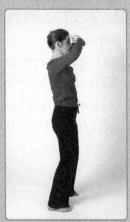
bring arms in, fingertips pointing to forehead

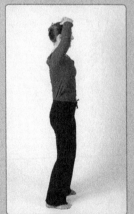
bring palms above the head

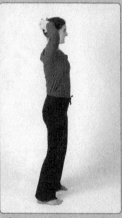
bring palms to the back of the head

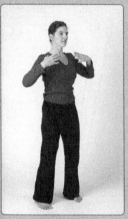
bring palms to the shoulders

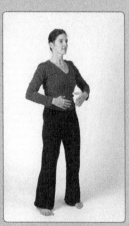
bring palms to belly

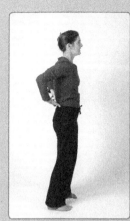 *bring palms to kidneys*

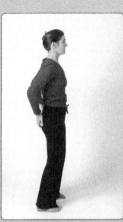 *bring palms to buttocks*

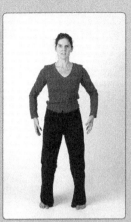 *bring palms to the side of legs*

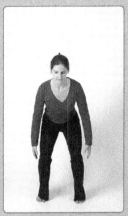 *bring palms to the side of knees*

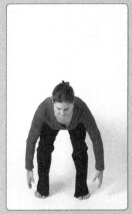 *bring palms to ankles*

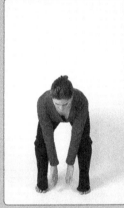 *at the level of the feet bring palms inside move them up the inner legs*

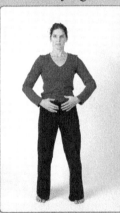 *place palms before lower belly and rest in dantian*

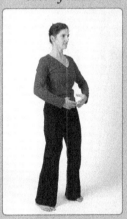 *start anew*

move in hands from lower belly to heart, forehead, head, shoulders, chest, belly, kidneys, outside of legs, inside of legs.

palms never touch the physical body, only the energy-body or jade body.

do as many cycle as you wish.

Example for a 15 to 20-minute work-out
1. » Warm-ups
2. » Four Essential Movements
   » Cleanse the Jade Body
5. » Wudang Qigong

3 standing
4 filling belly with chi

The Work-out

Qigong and Haiku

The old pond;
A frog jumps in:
Sound of water.
   Basho

> Once I stayed at a Zen Buddhist centre in France. There was a pond in the garden where I used to practice my qigong movements and postures. I had found a collection of haiku poetry in the in-house library which I took with me to read in the garden in between my qigong exercises.

Haiku poems date from 9th century Japan to the present day. Each haiku has three lines: the first line has 5 beats, or syllables, the second line has 7 beats, and the third has 5 beats. Haikus are usually inspired by nature, even though any thought or emotion can be expressed through this very compact form. A haiku is more than a type of poem; it is a way of looking at the physical world and seeing something deeper, like the very nature of existence. A single moment, movement or experience is captured in its entirety. Masters of ancient haiku poetry often spent their years in travelling, wandering, observing, contemplating and meditating, refining their craft into timeless literary flashes. Composing poems was a way to express their feeling and understanding of the ineffable power and mystery of life.

The haiku masters understood that the realities of life are most truly seen in everyday things and actions.
 They realised that our individual perceptions of worth, correctness, beauty, size and value are all relative and do not exist outside of ourselves.

They were aware that security and changelessness could never be found in nature and that acceptance of impermanence and opening to the unknown create a relaxing faith into the universe.

> *After I had looked at some of the poems I got up from the wooden bench next to the pond and returned to my practice, the images of the last haiku still reverberating in my mind. While I was adjusting myself in the standing posture I realised that something had changed. It felt like the distance between me and the natural environment had considerably lessened. Everything seemed close and clear and brilliant: the patches of bamboo behind the pond, the fishes in the water, the flowers in their beds. I understood that I was an integral part of the world surrounding me. Everything existed in relation to other things and everything was energetically connected.*
>
> *The haikus in conjunction with the qigong had caused a momentary internal shifting in the body-mind. It became clear to me that there was a striking congeniality between the two arts. Both came from the same greater cultural source and were pointing at the same essence. Their spirit was ultimately the same and their respective contemplative practices were intensifying the effect of each other.*

Qigong and the art of haiku are based on the creative tension between the contrasting elements of yin and yang, between stillness and movement, continuance and change, timelessness and time, humanity and nature.
In the perfect and relaxed interplay of yin and yang a greater harmony is achieved and a deeper life is touched.

Using Haiku Contemplation during a Qigong Session

Look for a suitable environment that facilitates your practice. Ideally it will be a spot in nature.

Let the "whirl" inside you gradually slow down.

Let the awareness go through your body, your posture and then expand it outside of yourself encompassing the environment.

If you are in nature look at the plants and trees; maybe there are stones or rocks, or some form of water, like a stream, a pool, a lake, or the sea. Look at the sky.

Now let a qigong exercise emerge out of yourself and sense the qi flowing through you.

When you feel ready, stop the exercise, take up the book and read the haiku poem(s) you have chosen once or twice. It's a tiny part of the panorama of life encapsulated in words.
    Let the image permeate you. Feel it with your whole body-mind.
    Feel the immediacy of the picture conveyed.

pond
frog
plop!

All happening in the same timeless moment

Can you feel yourself as a form that has come out of formless energy, out of qi? Can you just be aware like the pond, the water-lilies, the frog in a non-span of time?
    Can you see that all are parts of a functioning whole?

Qigong and Haiku

From that heightened sense of awareness, from the expansion of the body-mind, go back to your qigong exercise.

Your experience of qigong will be profound and extensive. Take this heightened quality of being into the activities of your life.

A selection of twelve haikus to contemplate

A cool breeze;
A whispering in the pines
Fills the air.
      Onitsura

On a leafless branch
Perched a crow:
An autumn eve.
      Basho

All creatures!!!
They squirm about among
The flowers in bloom.
      Issa

A mountain temple;
A monk's hand missed the bell!
A faint sound.
      Buson

Two butterflies:
They dance in the air till,
Double-white, they meet.
                    Basho

Above the mist veil
From time to time
The lake lifts a sail.
                    Basho

A frog!
Quietly and serenely
He gazes at the mountains.
                    Issa

The white chrysanthemum:
Not a speck of dust
To be seen.
                    Basho

A camellia dropped down
Into the water
Of a still, dark well.
      Buson

A raging sea!
Above Sado Island lies
The Milky Way.
      Basho

Surprise!
A snail at my feet.
When did it get here?
      Sokan

The skylark
Sings in the field:
Free of all things.
      Basho

CPSIA information can be obtained at www.ICGtesting.com
Printed in the USA
LVOW03s1915090514

385164LV00012B/211/P

THE CHEESEMAKING WORKSHOP

THE CHEESEMAKING WORKSHOP

WORKSHOP

Handmade cheeses and the beautiful
meals they create

LYNDALL DYKES

Contents

Introduction 07
Cheese 09
Cheese types 10
Starter cultures 12
Equipment 13
Methods explained 14

Blue vein	22
Bocconcini	32
Brie	38
Butter cultured	44
Camembert	49
Cheddar	55
Cheese curds	62
Edam	64
Fetta	68
Haloumi	76
Havarti	84
Kefir	88
Mascarpone	90
Monterey jack	96
Mozzarella	104
Paneer	110
Quark	114
Boursin	116
Ricotta	118
Romano	128
Washed rind	132
Yoghurt	138
Goat cheese	142
Affinage	148
Platter suggestions	150
Q & A	151
Tricks of the trade	153
Glossary	154
Index	156
Acknowledgements	159
About the author	159

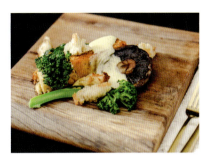
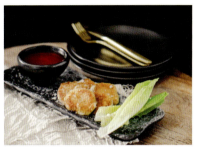
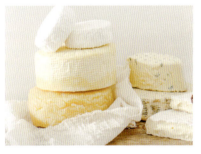
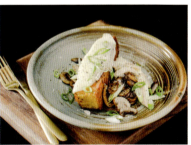
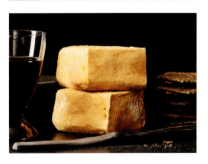

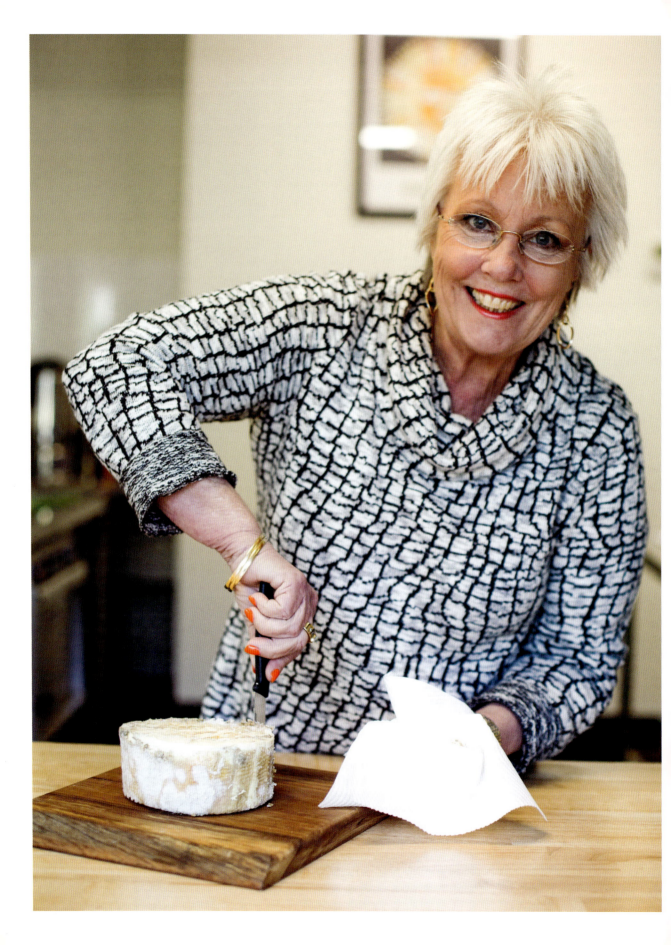

Introduction

It's my belief that if milkmaids can make cheese on a mountain plateau, with very little equipment as a way of preserving the milk for the winter months, then we can make it in our own kitchens. I'm always amazed at how dependent people have become on supermarkets. Cheese didn't originate in a plastic bag with a barcode on it—and with so many additives in it that you need a science degree to work out what it is you are eating.

You don't need to be an expert or a fantastic cook to create the basic foods we consume on a daily basis. All you need is some common sense and, of course, a little passion always helps.

In the following pages I will take the mystery out of making cheese, breaking it down into something that is so simple you will be able to create your own gourmet cheese at home.

My food journey started at a very young age. I became a vegetarian at fourteen and learnt the art of macrobiotic cooking at seventeen. I opened up a bulk health food shop with some friends at eighteen and taught vegetarian cooking at night school in my twenties. Food has always been a part of my life … I dream food, it inspires me. There are so many tangents to food that you can never stop learning about it.

After having children, a career and a few other distractions along the way, it was time to settle back into what I love most—food! And sharing a lifetime of acquired knowledge with people.

Being vegetarian, dairy has always been a part of my diet, so making cheese at home was just a natural thing to do. I get so excited about teaching people how to make cheese at home with so little equipment and now I just want to let everyone know how it is done!

How to use this book

It's important to know how to read through the recipes and know where help is when needed. Please take the time to read these pages before commencing your first cheese.

As you commence cheesemaking, you will find each step has photographic illustration as well as an explanation. If you need further information about any of the steps, please go to the **Methods Explained** section. If you require information on some of the cheese terminology, refer to the **Glossary** in the back of the book.

What to do with your cheese

There are many delicious cheese-inspired recipes featured in this book that will get your mouth watering! Of course, each cheese is amazing on its own—especially as you will be making it yourself.

I hope you enjoy this book as much as I have enjoyed putting it together!

Lyndall

www.thecheesemakingworkshop.com.au

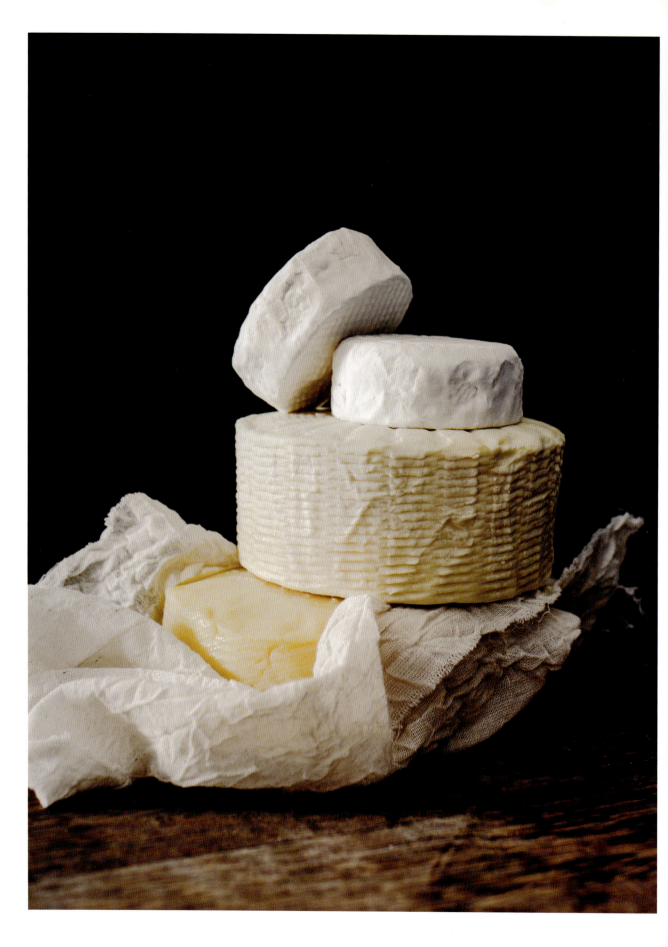

Cheese

Cheese is one of the most ancient forms of manufactured food. It even predates breadmaking. In fact, its origins predate recorded history.

The word 'cheese' comes from the Latin word caseus from which casein (milk protein) is derived.

It is thought cheesemaking dates back as early as 12,000BC. Evidence has been found in murals on the walls of tombs in Ancient Egypt, of cheese being buried with the pharaohs.

The Romans spread uniform cheesemaking techniques throughout Europe. Then with the collapse of the trade routes, cheesemaking became more diversified, each locality producing their own distinctive products. That is why so many cheeses are the same, but different. Like Brie and Camembert, the cheese takes on the name of the town or region in which it is made. The recipe is similar, the difference in the flavor comes from the different breeds of animals and the pastures on which the milking herds are feeding. The size, shape and maturing conditions also influence the final cheese.

In the mid 19th Century, a lot of cheesemaking went from farm gate to factories where it was mass produced and lost its individuality and quaintness. The next 100 years saw the decline of home cheesemaking. Now in the 21st Century, there is an increased interest in getting back to basics, in becoming more sustainable and producing your own food from scratch. With this new awareness in creating natural foods, boutique cheeseries are emerging all over the world producing stunning handmade cheeses.

We, as cheesemakers, can keep alive the ancient skills and traditions used for making a variety of cheese. Making cheese was a necessity and a skill that has survived thousands of years.

Let's get back to being a little more sustainable and take responsibility for the food we consume.

This book gives you step-by-step instructions on how to not only make your own beautiful cheese but also butter and yoghurt. Furthermore, it also gives you many delicious recipes in which to use your homemade cheese. It is satisfying knowing what is going into the food we make and that there are no preservatives or additives. It's also cost effective and when you present your homemade cheese to family and friends, the bragging rights are huge!

Cheese Types

There are so many different cheeses out there it is easy to get confused with what's what in terms of cheese types, so here's a little break down of what you can expect from each type without going overboard on detail.

Fresh cheeses These are cheeses that can be dolloped. A fresh cheese should not be sticky gooey or stretchy, they have no protective rind and are eaten fresh. Fresh cheeses include quark, mascarpone, crème fraîche and ricotta.

Soft cheeses
These are cheeses that, when at room temperature, can be cut with a butter knife. Their oozy delicious texture can be spread and are some of our favorite cheeses. Brie, camembert, chèvre, d'Affinois, blue cheese such as gorgonzola dolce and many washed rinds.

Semi hard cheeses
These are cheeses that dent when pressed firmly with a finger, but will spring back into shape. Familiar cheeses are Colby, some cheddars, Emmental, gouda, Havarti and some blues.

Hard cheeses
These are your parmesan, pecorinos, Romano, some cheddars and goudas.

Cheeses also come under more unfamiliar categories such as Fudgy. These are cheeses that are to firm to spread. These include some blues, Taleggio and Munster.

Crumbly
These are cheeses that will crumble, such as some fettas. Crumbly cheese will not become soft when at room temperature and will never be soft enough to spread.

Washed rind cheese
They are washed in a mild brine solution with Brevi linens, or they can be washed in beer or wine, I have also used Grand Manier! The washing process starts to happen a few days after the cheese is made and it really is as simple as giving the cheese a little bath, if brevi linens are used these creates a sticky often orange tinge to the rind of the cheese. The smell can be a little strong but the flavor is amazing.

Cheese can also be described as supple, flaky, stretchy and, of course, they all come under the one big category of **DELICIOUS**.

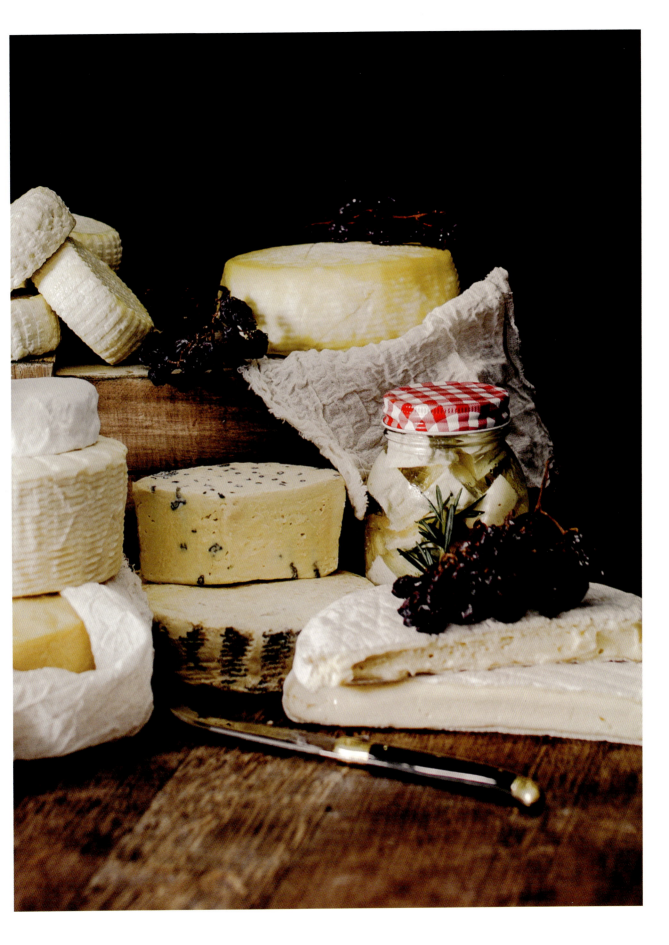

Starter Cultures

Up until the 1880s, the natural souring of the milk or sour whey from the previous day's cheesemaking was used as a starter. Today, we use blends of freeze-dried lactic bacteria or cultures to ensure we have a consistent product.

Choosing a starter to make your homemade cheese should not be a difficult thing to do, so let's simplify this. There are two main starters used in cheesemaking: Mesophilic and Thermophilic. We name ours 'Type M starter' for Mesophilic and 'Type T starter' for Thermophilic.

Having a basic understanding of how and why the cultures work will help you choose what you need. The purpose of the culture is to convert the lactose into lactic acid, to give your cheese its flavor and aroma. The culture puts the bacteria back into the milk that has been removed through pasteurisation. The culture will aid in preserving the cheese. The type M starter culture is used in cheese that is made at lower temperatures. Type M starter is the most commonly used starter and is used to make camembert, fetta, chèvre, blue vein, farmer house cheddar, cheddar, brie, quark, and many others. Type T starter is used in cheese made at higher temperatures such as parmesan, mozzarella, washed rind, mascarpone, to name a few.

Milk is a perfect medium for both good and bad bacteria to grow. The starter culture inoculates the milk with the good type of bacteria which multiply by consuming the lactose in the milk. This raises the acidity and once the good bacteria have taken hold in the milk, they help prevent the bad bacteria from gaining a foothold. Although the good bacteria from your M or T starter helps prevent any bad bacteria from appearing in your cheese, you still need to be vigilant about having a clean work area and utensils.

Mesophilic Culture = Type M Starter
(Lactococcus Lactis ssp cremoris)

This is used to make most of the cheeses in this book such as camembert, fetta, cheddar, havarti, quark, edam and more ...

Thermophilic Culture = Type T Starter
(Streptococcus Thermopholis)

This is used to make mozzarella, romano, washed rind and mascarpone.

Mesophilic Aromatic Starter = Type MA *(Flora Danica)*

This culture really gives the cheese a creamier texture with a buttery flavor. Such ideal cheeses include blue vein and our double cream brie. It also may be used in place of Type M starter.

ABY Probiotic Yoghurt Culture = Yoghurt Culture 1 *(Lactobacillus delbruecki subsp. bulgaricus)*

This is your typical Greek yogurt culture which has a sharp note at the end of the palate.

ABT Probiotic Yoghurt Culture = Yoghurt Culture 2 *(Lactobacillus acidophilus casei bifidobacterium)*

A little less tart than the other culture. Very child friendly.

Equipment

The equipment we use is as simple as the process itself.

- 15 litre (507 fl oz) styrene box to insulate our cheese vat
- Cheese vat—a 10 litre (338 fl oz) food grade container
- Curd turning spoon (you have to be careful you don't get your words mixed, when you say this). This is a slotted spoon
- Curd cutting knife (a pallet knife)
- Curd cutting rack (a cake cooling rack or similar)
- Thermometer (get a good digital one as temperature is important when making cheese)
- Mini measuring spoons—these are labelled a pinch, smidgen, tad, dash and drop
- Syringes to measure the rennet
- Cheese hoops
- Cheesecloth

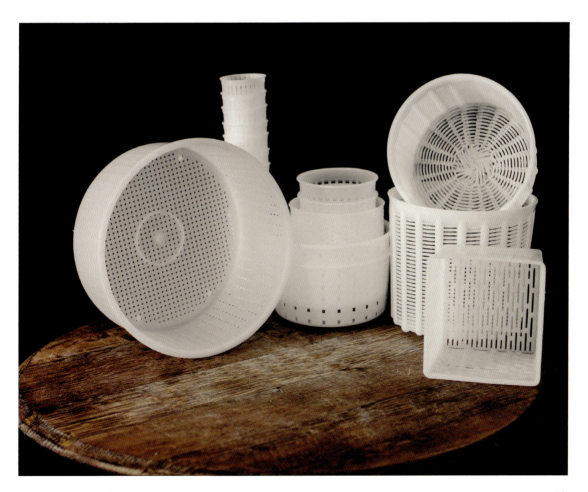

Methods Explained

Heating milk
Pour the milk, and addition of cream if the recipe requires it, into a saucepan and heat to the desired temperature. This will ensure the milk is warm enough to allow the culture to multiply, but not hot enough to adversely affect it.

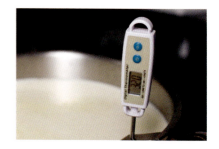

Adding Starter Culture
As we live in a time poor society, I am using the DVS (direct vat set) method for adding the starter. Simply add a small amount, usually a pinch spoon or $^1/_{10}$ of a teaspoon, of the specified freeze-dried culture sprinkled directly to the warm milk and stirring it through.

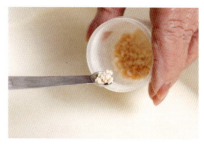

Cool pre-boiled water
If you are on town water, there will be chlorine in the water. Chlorine will kill the enzymes. All you need to do to remove the chlorine is bring the water to the boil and cool the water before using.

Adding Lipase
Lipase is an enzyme and must be diluted in cold pre-boiled water before adding to the milk.

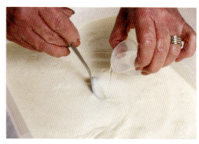

Adding rennet
The rennet we use is a microbial rennet—it is vegetarian. Rennet is an enzyme that sets the curd. The liquid rennet we use must be diluted in at least ten times its own volume of cold pre-boiled water and then poured over as much of the surface area of the milk as possible. It is then stirred through thoroughly to ensure you have an evenly set curd, approximately 30 seconds of stirring will do.

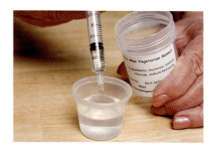

Adding mould spores
Adding white or blue mould spores to the milk is as easy as sprinkling the powder into the milk then stirring it through. A little goes a long way.

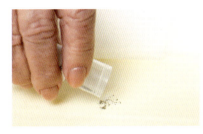

Resting the milk
This allows the cultures to multiply through the milk and gives the rennet time to set a curd. You need to maintain the starting temperature of the milk by insulating it for the required amount of time. We use a polystyrene box with the lid on.

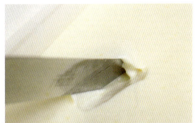

Checking the curd
To check the curd is ready to cut, place the blade of a knife or spatula into the curd on a 45-degree angle at 3 cm (1¼ inch) deep. Lift the knife blade to check the curd for a clean break. If it is a little soft, then let it rest for a further 10 minutes. If it hasn't set properly, please refer to the troubleshooting section of this book.

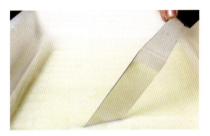

Cutting the curd
Cutting the curd is a term that refers to slicing the curd into cubes which creates a surface area for whey to be released. This is done by placing the blade of a knife or spatula into the curd at the desired width. (Each recipe will have a different width for the curd to be cut e.g. 1 cm, 2 cm ...) Slice the curd down the length of the box, then from left to right to create squares in the curd's appearance. After you have cut the curd in both directions, you will need to slide a curd rack through the curd with the lines of the rack horizontal. This will cut the curd into cubes. The size of the cut will determine the moisture content of the cheese. The smaller the cubes, the drier the cheese will be as more whey is released. The larger the cubes, the more moisture is retained in the curd creating a softer cheese.

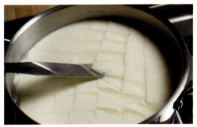

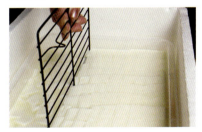

Turning the curd

As the curd is fragile to start with, you need to be gentle when first turning the curd. It isn't so much as a turning process, but more of a lift and jiggle! Place the slotted spoon as gently as you can down the side of the vat to the bottom of the tub. Then slowly and gently lift and jiggle the curd. This action encourages the whey to be released. As more whey is released and the curd firms up, you don't need to be quite as gentle.

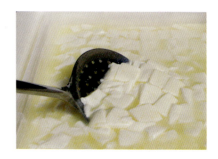

Draining the whey

To drain the whey from the curd, use a slotted spoon and a jug. The spoon should cover the opening of the jug. Gently submerge the jug with the slotted spoon, covering the opening into the curds and whey so the curd remains in the tub and the whey seeps through the spoon into the jug. You may need another jug on standby in case you need to measure how much whey you're removing. If you are draining the whey so that you can hoop the curd, then you remove as much of the whey as you can. Don't be tempted to pour the curd through a colander/sieve as it will break the curd up.

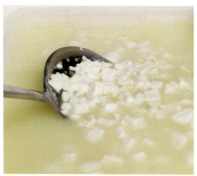

The word whey comes up all the time when draining whey and hooping curd.

We find so many songs with the word whey in them. Also lots of cheesy jokes:

Cheesemakers don't grow old, we just lose our whey!

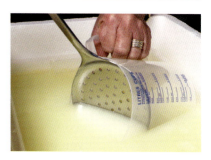

Cooking the curd. Method 1

Remove the required amount of whey as per recipe from the curd and replace with approximately the same amount of water at the specified temperature. This needs to be done slowly a little bit at a time. Slowly add a percentage of the water, checking the temperature and moving the curd around to distribute the warm water throughout the whole vat. Move hot spots to cold spots and vice versa so the temperature of the curd is even. Then continue to add small amounts of the remaining water into the curd whilst gently moving the curd and constantly checking the temperature until you have

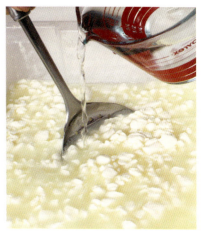

reached an all-over even temperature at the specified temperature. Be gentle, you don't want to break your curds up too much when cooking soft cheese curds for cheese like brie and camembert.

Cooking the curd. Method 2

This is the bain-marie method. This can be done depending on the instructions for the cheese you are making by either using a double-boiler or by placing water in-between the 10 litre (338 fl oz) cheese vat and the polystyrene box. When first turning the curd you will need to be gentle. As the curd firms up you don't need to be quite as gentle. If making a firm cheese, it helps to remove some of the whey during the turning and cooking process. This assists with reaching the desired temperature of the curd by not wasting energy on heating the whey. Be sure not to remove too much whey—you need it to help turn the curd.

Hooping the curd

Firstly, you will need to drain the whey away. Taking the curd turning spoon and a plastic jug, drain off as much of the whey as possible. Then using the curd turning spoon, place the curd into the hoops and fill each hoop to the top. Don't be tempted to go back and top up the cheese hoops until you have filled all the hoops to the same level, as the curd settles quickly. Once filled, the hoops need to be placed on a draining rack. Cover the hoops with cheesecloth and rest for 5 minutes. The hoops then need to be inverted—this is done by holding onto the cheesecloth and hoop and inverting it over onto the draining tray. When you need to turn it again, you simply hold onto the cheesecloth and invert the hoop back the other way, so the curd rests back in it. Make sure the cheese has settled into the very bottom of the hoop as this inverting is to give your cheese a nice shape. This needs to be done as per recipe. With every turn, you should remove any whey that is left in the tray.

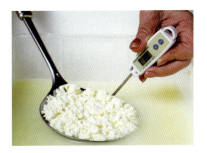
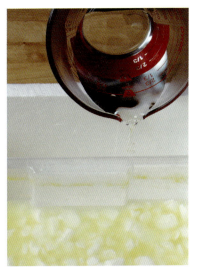
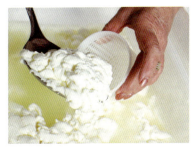
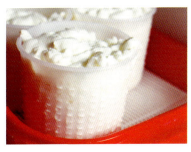

Brine solution

A brine solution is simply salt and water. Add the amount of non-iodised salt as per the recipe into an appropriate container, then fill it up with the required amount of boiling water. We use boiling water to help dissolve the salt but also boiling the water removes the chlorine. Use non-iodised salt when cheesemaking as iodine kills bacteria.

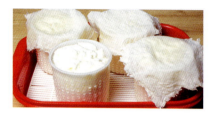

Brine bath

Some cheeses need to be bathed in brine (salt water). Choose a container that when the curd is sitting in the brine it comes halfway up the cheese. Place the set curd in the brine solution for the required time. Turn them over halfway through the brining to make sure all surfaces are brined. Some cheese is washed in brined with an added ingredient. Simply make your brine solution as per recipe then add brevi linens to the brine as per the recipe. Brine helps with the flavor of the cheese and slows the cheese maturation process down.

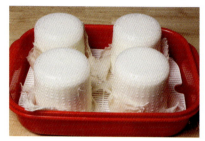

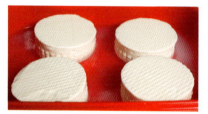

Salting the curd

Some cheese curds are salted before hooping; this is a matter of putting the non-iodised salt into the cheese curd once the whey has been removed, then gently folding it through. Try the curd, if it is not salty enough add a little more, but remember to add the salt is small amounts. You can always add more but once in, you can't remove it. Other cheeses are rubbed with salt. Remove the set, shaped curd from the hoop—they should be firm and you will be able to pick it up easily. Using non-iodised salt, rub the cheese all over with the suggested amount of salt as per recipe.

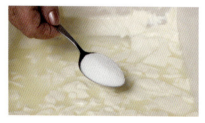

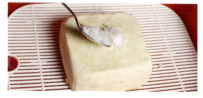

Storing cheese in brine

Some cheese such as fetta and haloumi have no salt added to the curd but are stored in a brine. Make the brine solution to the recipe and place the curd into the brine. Make sure they are completely submerged. To store them, place in the fridge.

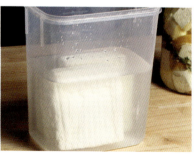

Piercing the cheese (blue vein)
Using a thermometer probe or thin knitting needle, pierce the cheese from the top to the bottom at the suggested intervals as per recipe. You can pierce it through from left to right all the way around. The more holes you create, the more, blue veins the cheese will develop.

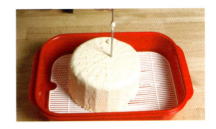

Cleaning the cheese (blue vein)
Some cheeses don't present very well. To make your cheese more presentable, scrape the surface mould off using a paring knife. Scrape along the top, bottom and sides of the cheese to take off excess mould growth. This is done with blue vein after maturation, just before wrapping the cheese and placing it in the fridge.

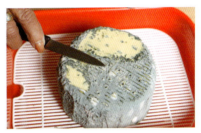

Cheddaring curd
To cheddar the curd allow the curd to knit together when they have formed a slab cut into chunks and stack onto of each other to remove more whey.

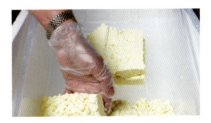

Chipping or milling the curd (cheddar)
This can be done in two ways: Cutting the curd into rectangular shapes (chips) or breaking up the curd with your hands, before salting.

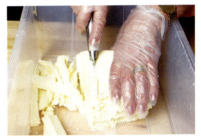

Washing the curd
Certain cheeses need water added to the curd to wash lactic acid from their curd. Add water at the required temperature to the curd as per recipe instructions.

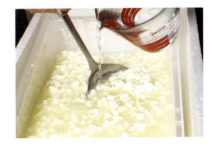

Maturation for surface ripened cheese

With camembert and brie, we inoculate the milk with a *Penicillium Candidum* or more commonly called, white mould spore. Although we add the white mould spore into the milk, mould needs air to grow and form the rind on the surface of the cheese. To achieve this, you will need to create a humid environment at a controlled temperature of between 10–15°C (50°–59°F). Essentially we are trying to recreate a cave. How we create this humid environment is by simply placing the lid on a draining rack container. The lid must not touch the cheese as this will inhibit any mould from growing. While it's at this stage, the cheese will need to be turned over every day to ensure the mould bloom grows evenly over the cheese—be sure to wipe out any excess moisture. Turning everyday also prevents the mould from growing around the bottom of the racks and attaching itself.

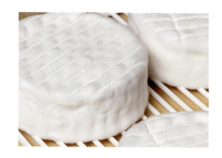

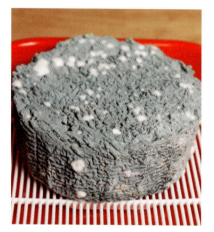

Keeping the cheese at 10°–15°C (50°–59°F) is easy if you have a wine fridge. Just place the whole container in the wine fridge and turn the cheese every day. If you don't have a wine fridge or cellar, you will need to keep the cheese in their containers with the lids on inside the polystyrene box or esky (cooler) with a frozen ice brick. You will need to change the ice-brick morning and night so you will need to have two ice-bricks on hand. Once the cheese has an even coverage of mould, usually around 8–10 days, wrap, date* and place in the regular fridge at 4°C (39°F).

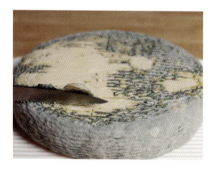

* Date written is the day cheese was made.

Waxing the cheese

Waxing is a very rewarding part of cheesemaking. It makes the finished product look professional and appealing. Traditional colors are used on certain cheeses which helps identify the cheese you make so they don't need to be labelled. The wax is essential to make an airtight barrier.

To wax the cheese, simply purchase a block of food grade cheese wax and place it in a saucepan you won't

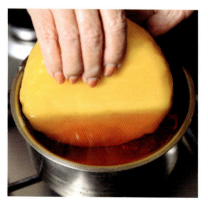

need to use again (you can usually pick up something cheap at charity shop).

Heat the wax on a medium temperature until it has just melted. Cool your cheese down by placing it in the fridge for a few hours—it will make it much easier to handle. Dip the cheese into the melted wax (halfway up the cheese) then hold it up so the drips run down the coated side until it is dry. Change your grip so you are now holding the waxed side and dip the uncoated side into the wax. Hold it up to dry and repeat this process so the wax is evenly coated three times. The wax can be stored in the wax saucepan and reheated to use again. Discard the old wax when removing it from the cheese.

Another option is to cryovac the cheese.

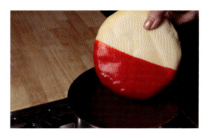

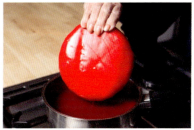

Blue Vein

The Italians are renowned for their gorgonzola, the English for their stilton and the French for their roquefort. Each type of blue cheese has its own characteristic, but they all share a common network of blue veins throughout the cheese. My blue is made from non-homogenised milk and has one semi-soft texture with a flavor that's not too strong. The other is a firmer stilton style. The flavor differs with age so if you like a stronger blue cheese, leave it for a few more weeks than our recipe suggests.

The legend behind the original roquefort cheese is that it came into existence by accident... A young and lustful shepherd stowed his lunch in a nearby cave and at the promise of a kiss, abandoned his flock and his lunch, which was in the cave, to pursue a pretty maiden that happened by. He returned three days later (long kiss) to find his cheese had grown a blue/green coat! Hungry, the shepherd ate his cheese and found it to be noticeably delicious!

Creamy Blue

A soft double cream blue vein

Makes 600 g (1 lb 5 oz)

4 litres (135 fl oz/16 cups) non-homogenised milk
200 ml (7 fl oz) pure cream
1 pinch spoon type MA culture
1 speck blue mould spore
1.2 ml (0.04 fl oz) liquid vegetarian rennet
20 ml (½ fl oz) boiled water, cooled
1 tablespoon non-iodised salt

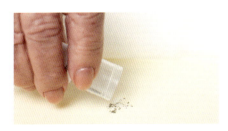

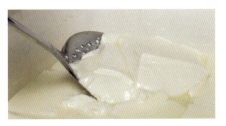

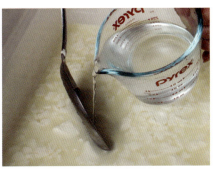

Day 1

In a large saucepan, heat the non-homogenised milk and pure cream to 35°C (95°F). Once warmed, transfer the milk to your cheese vat. To your milk, add the type MA culture and stir thoroughly. Add a very fine sprinkle of the blue mould spore to the milk and mix thoroughly. Mix the liquid vegetarian rennet with the cold, pre-boiled water. Pour the diluted rennet immediately into the milk, taking care to pour it over as much of the surface as possible. Mix in well and allow the milk to set into a curd. This will take 1 hour.

Cut the curd

To check the curd, place the blade of a knife into the curd and lift at a 45-degree angle, looking for a clean break. If the curd parts well, it is ready to cut. Cut the curd in 3 cm (1¼ inch) intervals using a curd-cutting knife. Cut from top to bottom and left to right. Next, using a curd cutting rack to cut through horizontally. Allow curd to rest for 5 minutes.

Turn the curd

Using a curd-turning spoon, slide the spoon down the side of the vat and underneath the curd. Then gently lift and jiggle, bringing the spoon to the surface. Continue until all of the curd has been turned once. The curd will need to be turned every 10 minutes for the next hour.

Wash the curd

Taking a curd-turning spoon and a plastic jug, drain off 1 litre (35 fl oz/4 cups) whey. Wash the curd by replacing the 1 litre (35 fl oz/4 cups) whey with water at 30–33°C (86–91°F). Turn the curd gently for 5 minutes, then allow the curd to rest. Taking a curd-turning spoon and a plastic jug again, drain off as much of the whey as possible and sprinkle the curd with 1 level tablespoon of non-iodised salt. Gently stir the salt through the curd.

Using your curd-turning spoon again, ladle the curd into a 1 kg (2 lb 4 oz) cheese hoop and cover with a piece of cheesecloth. Allow the cheese to rest for 5 minutes. Invert the cheese hoop by holding onto the cheesecloth and turning the hoop over. Continue to invert hoops five times over the next 3 to 4 hours, remove whey as you go.

Leave the cheese in the hoop overnight at room temperature.

Day 2
The next morning, remove the cheese from the hoop and rub with a small amount of non-iodised salt. Leave the cheese to rest for 24 hours on a draining rack.

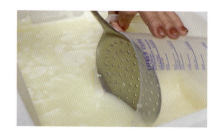

Day 3
Repeat the process of rubbing the surface of the cheese with a small amount of non-iodised salt. Leave the cheese to rest for 24 hours on a draining rack.

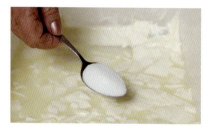

Day 4
Using your thermometer as a skewer, pierce right through the cheese at 1 cm (½ inch) intervals. This creates a network of veins for the blue mould to grow throughout the cheese. Place the lid on the draining rack container to create a humid environment and store your blue cheese at 10–15°C (50–59°F) for 12–14 days. You will see blue mould developing on the outside of your cheese in this time.

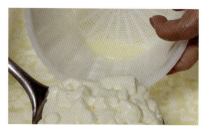

Once you see a good blue mould growth, chill the cheese in the fridge until it is easy to handle. Scrape the blue rind off your cheese using a sharp knife. This will create a slightly softer flavor and will present a better-looking cheese. Please note this step is completely optional and is not essential to your cheesemaking. Wrap your cheese in baking paper, then foil and store in your fridge at 4°C (39.2°F).

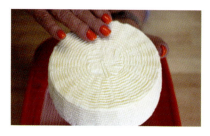

Notes:
This blue can be eaten from 1 month from the day it's made. Keep in mind that they will get a stronger flavor with age. To serve your homemade blue vein, remove the cheese from the fridge an hour before consuming. It is best served at room temperature.

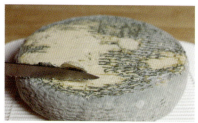

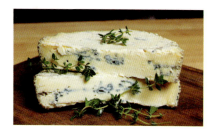

Stilton-Style Blue
A rich, slightly salty firm blue vein

Makes 600 g (1 lb 5 oz)

4 litres (135 fl oz/16 cups) non-homogenised milk
200 ml (7 fl oz) pure cream
1 pinch spoon type MA culture
1 speck blue mould spore
1 ml (0.03 fl oz) liquid vegetarian rennet
20 ml (½ fl oz) boiled water, cooled
1 tablespoon non-iodised salt

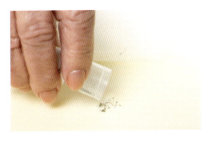

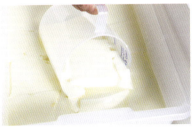

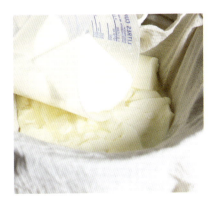

Day 1
In a large saucepan, heat the non-homogenised milk and pure cream to 30°C (86°F). Once warmed, transfer the milk to your cheese vat. Add the type MA starter. Add a very fine sprinkle of the blue mould spore to the milk and mix thoroughly. Leave for 45 minutes. Mix the liquid vegetarian rennet with the cooled boiled water. Pour diluted rennet immediately into the milk, taking care to pour it over as much of the surface as possible. Mix in well and allow the milk to set into a curd. This will take 1.5 hours.

Cut the curd
To check the curd is ready to cut, place the blade of a knife into the curd and lift at a 45-degree angle, looking for a clean break. If the curd parts well, it is ready to cut. Cut the curd at 5 cm (2 inch) intervals using a curd-cutting knife. Cut from top to bottom and left to right. Next, using a curd cutting rack to cut through horizontally. Allow curd to rest for 10 minutes.

Using a small jug, gently transfer the curd into a cheesecloth-lined colander. This should be stood over a saucepan or similar as the whey that drains from the curd will help to keep the curd warm. Leave the curd to sit for a further 1.5 hours. Remove the colander from the whey and allow the curd to drain until only a little whey is dripping out. Gather the cheesecloth together to form a bag and place a weight of about 4 kg (8 lb 13 oz) on top and leave it pressing overnight.

Day 2
The next morning, remove from cheese cloth and break the curd into 2.5 cm (1 inch) size pieces and sprinkle with the non-iodised salt and gently mix in. Place the curd into a 1 kg (2 lb 4 oz) cheese hoop and press for 30

minutes with approximately 6 kg (13 lb 3 oz) weights. Invert to give the cheese a nice shape, then press again maintaining pressure for 24 hours.

Day 3

Remove from hoop. Pierce holes at 1 cm (½ inch) intervals, right through the cheese. Place in maturation tray with the lid on and mature the cheese at 10–15°C (50–59°F) for between 4–8 weeks, turning every 4–5 days.

When the blue mould starts to break down, it will turn a brown color and become soft under the surface. Your cheese is now matured! Scrape any sticky brown mould from the cheese and wrap in baking paper, then foil. It is ready to consume now or can be stored for a further few weeks in the fridge. Remember the longer you leave it the stronger it will be.

Note

This cheese is best served at room temperature.

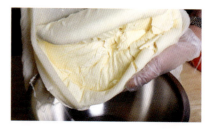
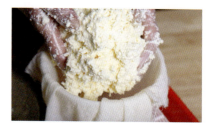
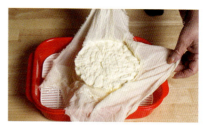
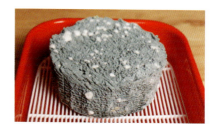
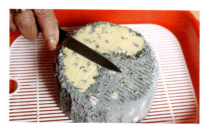
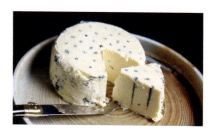

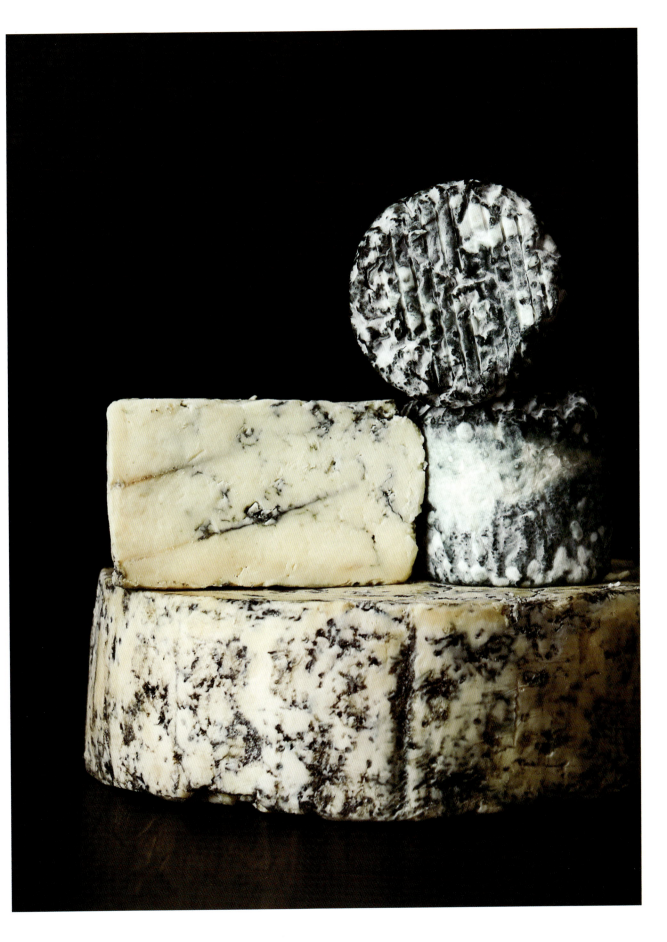

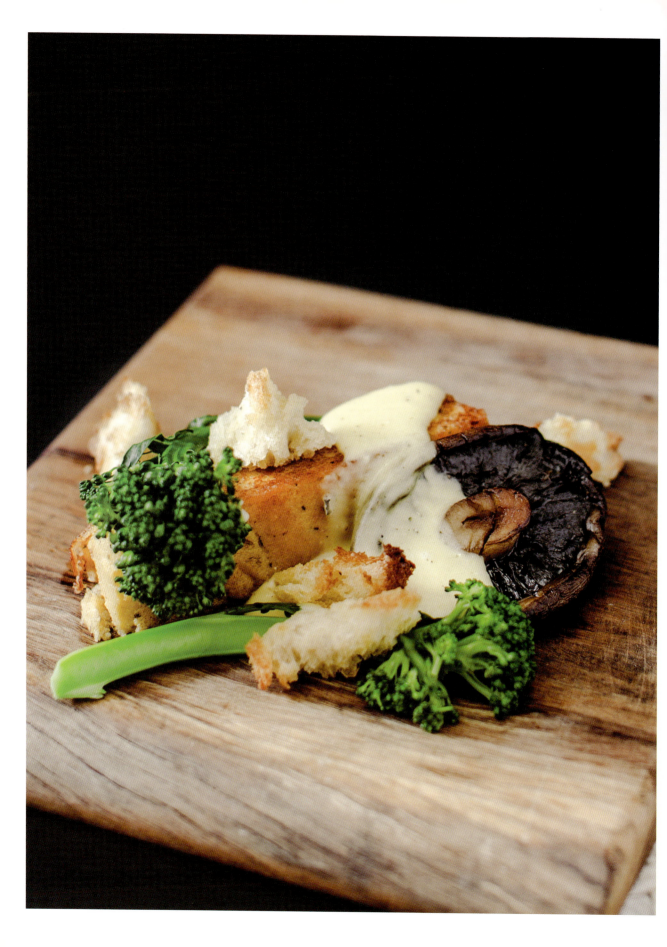

Portobello Mushrooms with Blue Cheese & Sourdough Croutons

Serves 6

Polenta
250 g (9 oz) polenta
1 litre (35 fl oz/4 cups) vegetable stock
50 g (1¾ oz) butter
125 g (4½ oz) grated parmesan cheese
rice bran oil, for frying

Sourdough Croutons
250 g (9 oz) sourdough bread
75 ml (2¼ fl oz) olive oil

Blue Cheese Sauce
1 garlic clove
250 g (9 oz) creamy blue cheese
150 g (5½ oz) mascarpone
salt and pepper, to season

6 portobello mushrooms
1 bunch broccolini
butter, for frying

To make the polenta, in a heavy-based saucepan, combine the polenta with enough cold water to dampen the polenta. Leave for 5 minutes. Bring the vegetable stock to the boil and slowly add to the cold polenta. Bring to the boil, stirring constantly as it will spit at you! Reduce the heat and cook for 5 minutes. Add the butter and parmesan. Place the hot polenta in a 20 cm x 20 cm (8 inch x 8 inch) baking dish. When cool, refrigerate for 1 hour or overnight.

To make the sourdough croutons, remove the crust from the bread and tear into small almond-sized pieces. Toss in the oil and bake until crisp. Set aside.

To make the blue cheese sauce, rub a small frying pan with the garlic and place half of the blue cheese and all of the mascarpone into the pan. Heat until melted and smooth, then season with salt and pepper to taste.

Pan-fry the mushrooms with the butter until soft. Blanch the broccolini in hot water for 2 minutes, then refresh under cold running water.

Slice the polenta into desired shapes and fry in a little oil until golden. Divide the polenta evenly onto six serving plates. Top with a mushroom and broccollini, then drizzle with blue sauce and scatter with croutons and remaining blue cheese.

Potato Gnocchi with Blue Cheese Sauce

Serves 4

The word gnocchi in Italian means 'little lump'. It was originally served as an extra during a traditional Italian meal. Gnocchi should be anything but lumpish as a well-made gnocchi should be light and fluffy. This recipe requires no egg—this helps to make the gnocchi light.

Gnocchi
500 g (1 lb 2 oz) désirée potatoes
250 g (9 oz) plain (all-purpose) flour

Sauce
20 g (¾ oz) butter
20 g (¾ oz) plain (all-purpose) flour
125 ml (4 fl oz) milk, heated to 90°C (194°F)
125 g (4½ oz) blue cheese
2 tablespoons mascarpone
freshly ground black pepper and salt, to season
grated parmesan cheese, to serve
chives, to garnish

Wash the potatoes and place in a large pot of cold water. Bring to the boil and cook until tender. Do not to pierce potatoes until you need to see if they are cooked through, as this will cause them to absorb water.

Drain the potatoes and peel them while they are still hot. Pass them through a potato ricer. Gradually add most of the flour to the potato, reserving a little. Knead into a smooth mixture.

Once the mixture becomes soft and smooth, stop kneading. Dust the work area with a little flour. Divide the mixture into four parts and roll into a sausage. If the gnocchi dough breaks and cracks, add more flour and knead until combined. Roll again into a sausage, cut into 1 cm (1/2 in) pieces and roll each piece down a gnocchi board. This creates a surface for the sauce to stick to the gnocchi.

Bring a saucepan of water to the boil. Place half the gnocchi into the boiling water, do not overcrowd the pot. Allow them to bob around in the pot. When they all rise to the surface, remove with a slotted spoon. Place them in an oiled dish, again don't overcrowd, and continue cooking remaining gnocchi.

To make the sauce, in a small saucepan, melt the butter, add the flour and stir until flour is totally covered in butter. Continue cooking and stirring for approximately 1 minute, then very slowly add the hot milk, stirring constantly. When the sauce becomes thick and smooth add the blue cheese and mascarpone. Do not boil. Season with salt and pepper.

Gently toss the gnocchi through the sauce. Garnish with parmesan and chives.

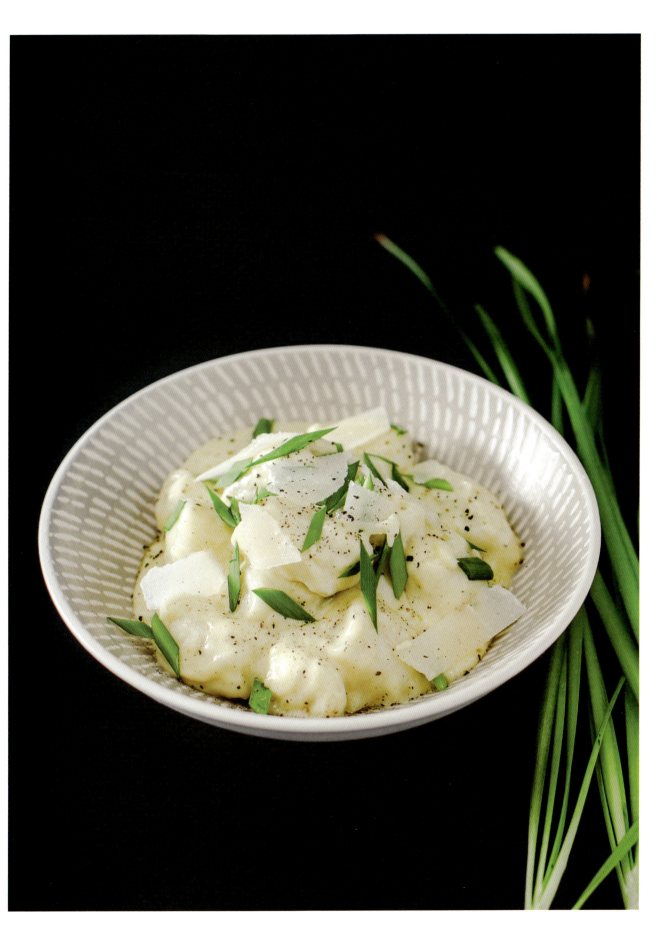

Bocconcini

Bocconcini is a small, fresh, semi-soft, white, mild cheese that originated in Naples and was made from the milk of water buffalos. Nowadays, it is often made from a combination of buffalo and cow's milk or straight cow's milk. Bocconcini from buffalo milk is now being produced in Australia since the introduction of buffalo dairies around the continent. This recipe for bocconcini is a bit of a cheat's version—it's a quick 15-minute microwave recipe. Not traditional but a bit of fun! It saves a trip to the shops on a Friday night when putting together those last-minute pizzas. You'll need a saucepan, microwave-safe bowl and rubber gloves. The cooking times are based on a 1000w microwave.

Bocconcini

Small egg sized shapes of mozzarella

Makes approximately 250 g (9 oz)

2 litres (70 fl oz/8 cups) non-homogenised milk
1 teaspoon citric acid
1 ml (0.03 fl oz) liquid vegetarian rennet
20 ml (½ fl oz) boiled water, cooled

Pour the milk into a saucepan and heat over high heat until it reaches 30°C (80°F). Add the citric acid and stir whilst heating the milk gently to 41°C (105.8°F). The milk should look a little textured.

Add the rennet to cold pre-boiled water and pour into the milk. Stir thoroughly. Allow the milk to set. This will take 5 minutes.

Scoop out the set curd with a slotted spoon and put it into a microwave-safe container. Microwave on high for 1 minute.

Using rubber gloves, knead the curd for approximately 30 seconds to release some whey. Drain off the whey. Place back into the microwave on high for 30 seconds. Knead the curd to release some more whey. Place back into the microwave on high for 30 seconds. The curd should now be melted and ready to stretch.

Stretch and fold the curd seven times. Then squeeze the curd through a closed fist to form little balls, or roll the curd into a sausage shape and slice into small bite-size portions. Place into a container of cold water to set, then remove from the water.

You can use it immediately or place it into a brine solution for approximately 1 hour and store in the fridge until ready to use. It will only keep for a few days, but is best to use the cheese as soon as it is made.

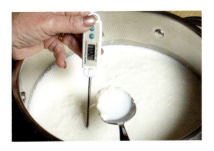

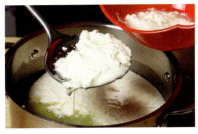

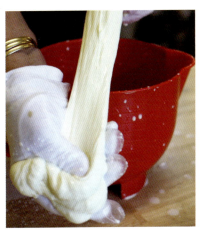

Crumbed Bocconcini

Serves 4 as an entrée

1 batch of bocconcini cheese
2 eggs, lightly beaten
250 g (9 oz) breadcrumbs
oil, for shallow-frying

Place the bocconcini balls into a bowl of lightly beaten eggs, then roll in the breadcrumbs. Repeat this method to double crumb for extra crunch!

Heat the oil in a frying pan over medium to high heat. Shallow pan-fry the balls, in batches, for approximately 4 minutes turning regularly, to brown on all surfaces, or until golden brown. Serve immediately with your favorite sauces.

Note

I love these little bocconcini balls with my home made capsicum sauce, but you could use sweet chilli, or even a little caramelized balsamic to dip them in. They look really pretty served on a bed of rocket and can also be served as a finger food or addition to tapas.

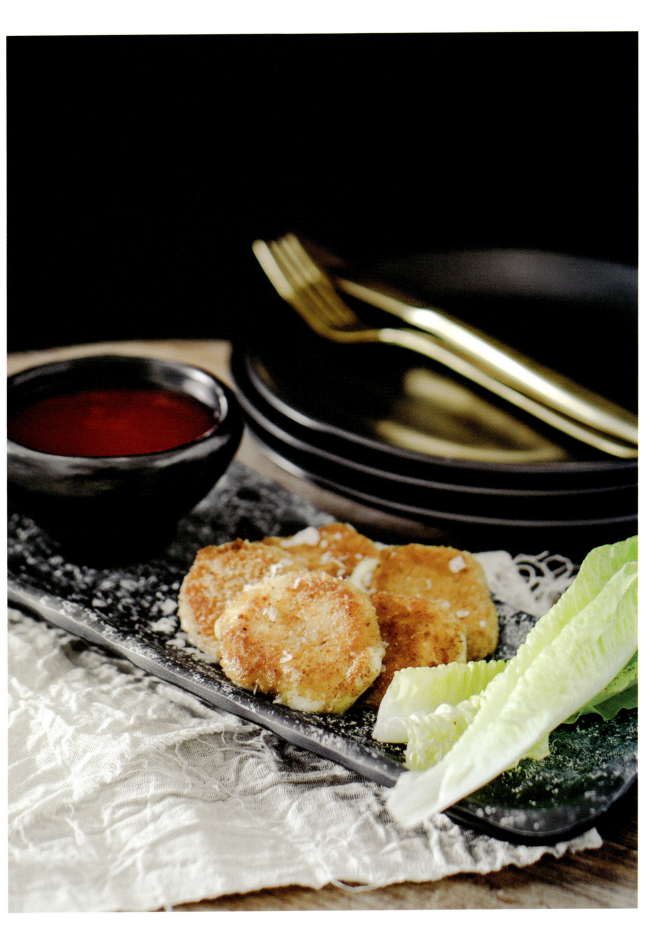

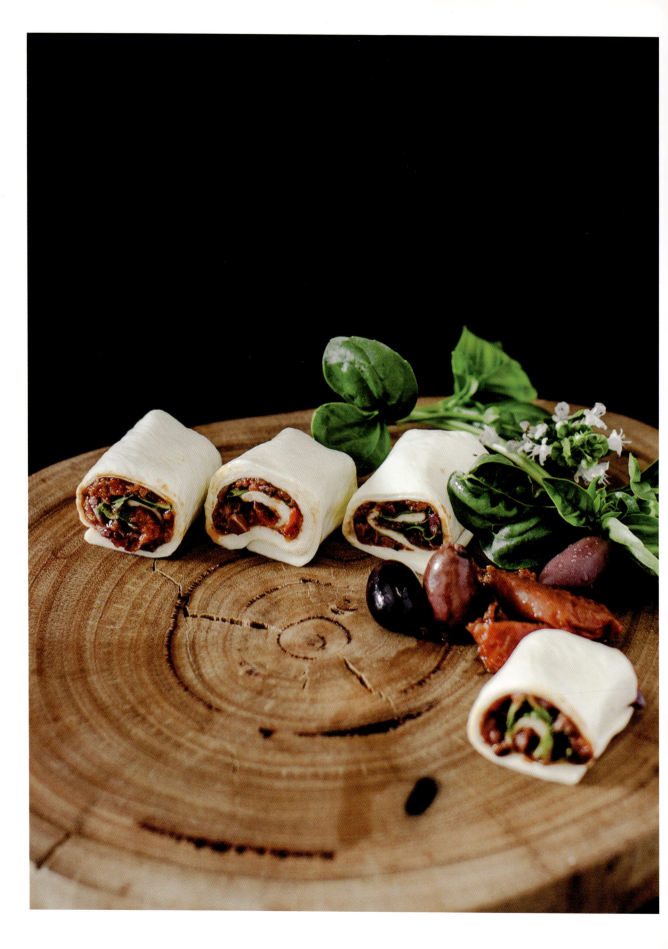

Bocconcini Pin Wheels

Serves 4 as an entrée

1 batch of bocconcini cheese
50 g (1¾ oz) tomato tapenade
50 g (1¾ oz) basil leaves, torn
2 tablespoons kalamata olives, finely chopped

Make the bocconcini as per recipe until you have finished stretching, then rather than making balls, spread the bocconcini out into a flat rectangle.

Spread with the tomato tapenade, sprinkle with the olives and basil and roll up like a Swiss roll.

Slice the roll into 2 cm (1 inch) rounds. Refrigerate until needed. Serve as an entrée or part of an antipasto platter.

Note
These are best eaten on the day they are made, or can they be stored in the fridge for a few days.

Brie

This gorgeous, buttery and earthy cheese was first created in the Middle Ages by the monks of the Priory of Rueil en Brie. It's reputation for being known as the cheese of kings began in 774 when the French Emperor stopped at the priory and discovered the cheese. Today, brie is enjoyed around the world, but I must say I do feel a little royal when I serve my own double cream brie, especially with the addition of fresh truffle.

Brie

A mild, creamy, double cream Brie

Makes 600 g (1 lb 5 oz)

4 litres (135 fl oz/16 cups) non-homogenised milk
160 ml (5¼ fl oz) pure cream
1 pinch spoon type MA type starter
2 drop spoons white mould spore
1.2 ml (0.04 fl oz) liquid vegetarian rennet
20 ml (½ fl oz) boiled water, cooled
100 g (3½ oz) non-iodised salt

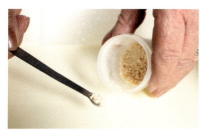

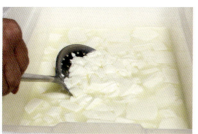

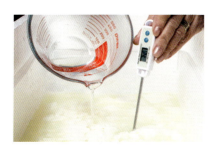

Day 1

In a large saucepan, heat the milk and pure cream to 32°C (89°F). Once warmed, transfer the milk to your cheese vat. To your milk, add the type MA starter, then one drop of the white mould spore and mix well. Leave for 1.5 hours.

Mix the liquid vegetarian rennet with the cold, pre-boiled water. Pour the diluted rennet immediately into the milk, taking care to pour it over as much of the surface as possible. Mix in well and allow the milk to set into a curd. This will take 40 minutes. Boil the jug, as you will need water at 60°C (140°F) to cook the curd in a later step.

Cut the curd

To check the curd, place the blade of a knife into the curd and lift at a 45-degree angle, looking for a clean break. If the curd parts well, it is ready to cut. Cut the curd in 3cm (1¼ inch) intervals using a curd cutting knife. Cut from top to bottom and left to right. Next, using a curd cutting rack, cut through horizontally. Allow curd to rest for 5 minutes.

Turn the curd

Using a curd turning spoon, slide the spoon down the side of the vat and underneath the curd. Then gently lift and jiggle, bringing the curd turning spoon to the surface. Continue until all of the curd has been turned once. Rest the curd for 10 minutes and gently turn again. Rest the curd again for another 10 minutes and turn again. The curd will need to be turned three times total.

Cooking the curd

Using a curd turning spoon and a plastic jug, place the curd turning spoon over the mouth of the jug and press into the curd gently to drain off 1 litre (35 fl oz/4 cups) whey and replace it with 1 litre (35 fl oz/4 cups) water from the previously boiled jug. If the curd is at 30°C (86°F) the temperature of your water should be at 60°C (140°F). Add the water slowly, bringing the temperature of the curd up to 34°C (93.2°F), maximum of 35°C (95°F). Make sure the temperature of the curd is even throughout the vat. Allow the curd to rest for 10 minutes.

Draining the whey

Taking a curd turning spoon and a plastic jug again, drain off as much of the whey as possible using the previous method. Then using a curd turning spoon, ladle the curd into a 1 kg (2 lb 4 oz) cheese hoop, filling to the top. Once filled, the hoop needs to be placed onto a draining tray. Cover the hoop with cheesecloth and rest for 5 minutes. Invert the hoop by holding onto the cheesecloth and turning over. Continue to invert the hoop five times over the next 3 to 4 hours and drain off any excess whey as you go.

Leave the curd in the hoop overnight at room temperature. Make your brine solution ready for tomorrow morning by adding the non-iodised salt, dissolved in 600 ml (21 fl oz) boiling water in a container that will have the brine solution halfway up the cheese. Leave overnight.

Day 2

The next morning, add the remaining drop spoon of white mould spore to brine solution and stir. Remove the cheese from the hoop and place into the cooled brine solution. Leave the cheese for 30 minutes, turn over, then leave for another 30 minutes. Remove the cheese from the brine solution and place on a draining rack for 24 hours to 48 hours at room temperature with no lid on. Turn the cheese every 12 hours to make sure it dries evenly, removing any whey from the draining rack container. Once your cheese feels clammy, not wet, place the lid on to the drying rack container to create a humid environment. Store the cheese between 10–15°C (50–59°F) for 8 to 10 days. The cheese needs to be turned every day. At day 4 the cheese will have started to grow a white mould on the exterior, this becomes the rind. After 8 to 10 days, your cheese will be covered with a bloom of white mould. Wrap your cheese in foil and store in the fridge at 4°C (39.2°F). The cheese should be ready to eat after 4 weeks from the day it was made.

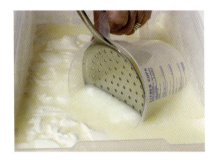
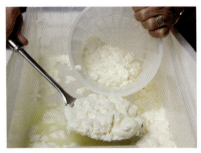
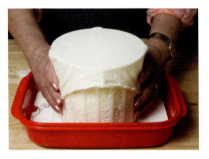
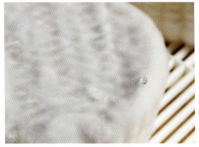
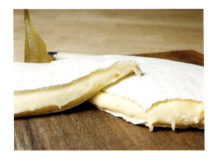

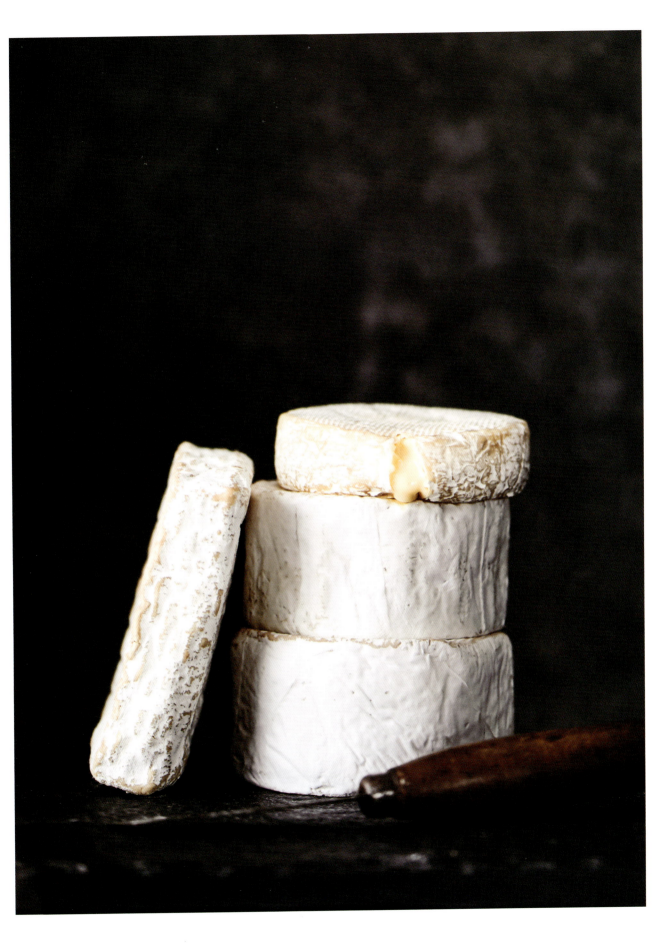

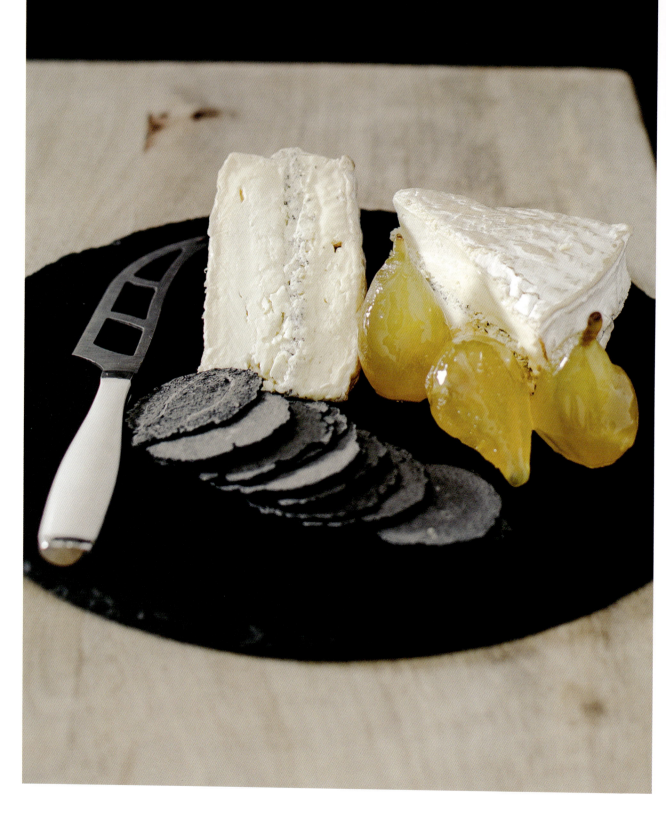

Truffle Brie

Serves 15–20

2 x 600 g (1 lb 5 oz) wheels of brie
150 g (5½ oz) mascarpone
10 g (¼ oz) freshly grated truffle
pinch of salt

Slice the top of both wheels of brie.

Mix the grated truffle with the mascarpone and season with a little salt. Spread the truffle mascarpone over the open side of one of the wheels of brie. Place the other brie on top, open side down, and smooth around the edges.

Now you have a huge homemade truffle brie to share with friend and family!

Butter Cultured

People have been making their own butter for centuries. Recorded uses of butter date back as far as 2000 years BC. In the past, home butter-making took time and energy, but even then, you only needed simple equipment. After the cows were milked, the milk was left to settle in a cool place so the cream would rise to the top, then the cream was skimmed off and put into a churn. The churning process was very labour intensive.

Moving the cream constantly is the churning process that actually produces butter, which sees the separating of the yellow fat from the buttermilk. Simply shaking cream in a jar will eventually turn it into butter.

Today, our job is made much easier with a mixer!

Butter Cultured

Makes approximately 250 g (9 oz) butter and 250 ml (9 fl oz) buttermilk

500 ml (17 fl oz) pure cream
1 pinch ABT probiotic culture
5 g (⅛ oz) salt (optional)

Pour the cream into a mixing bowl. Add the ABT probiotic culture and set aside for 4 hours. Once cultured, add in the salt.

Using the whisk attachment on an electric mixer, whip the cream on medium speed. It will thicken and become stiff then separate into butter and buttermilk. The butter will collect on the whisk. Line a sieve with cheesecloth, place it over a bowl and tip the butter and buttermilk into the cheesecloth-lined sieve. Scrape the butter off the whisk using a spatula.

Gather the cheesecloth around the butter to form a bag, then rinse the butter under cold running water until the water runs clear, then gently squeeze the excess water out.

Keep refrigerated in an airtight container and use within 14 days, or freeze for up to a month.

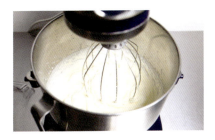
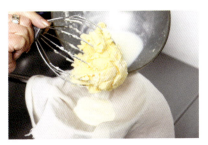
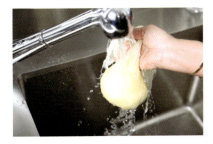
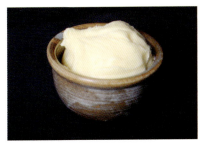

Truffle Butter

Makes 2 x 125 g (4½ oz) logs

250 g (9 oz) homemade butter, softened
20 g (¾ oz) finely grated truffle
sea salt, to taste

Mix all ingredients together in a bowl. Place half of the ingredients on a piece of plastic wrap. Shape the butter into a log about 5 cm (2 inches) in diameter. Wrap the log in plastic. Repeat with the remaining butter.

The butter will keep in the fridge for a week, or can be stored for up to a month in the freezer.

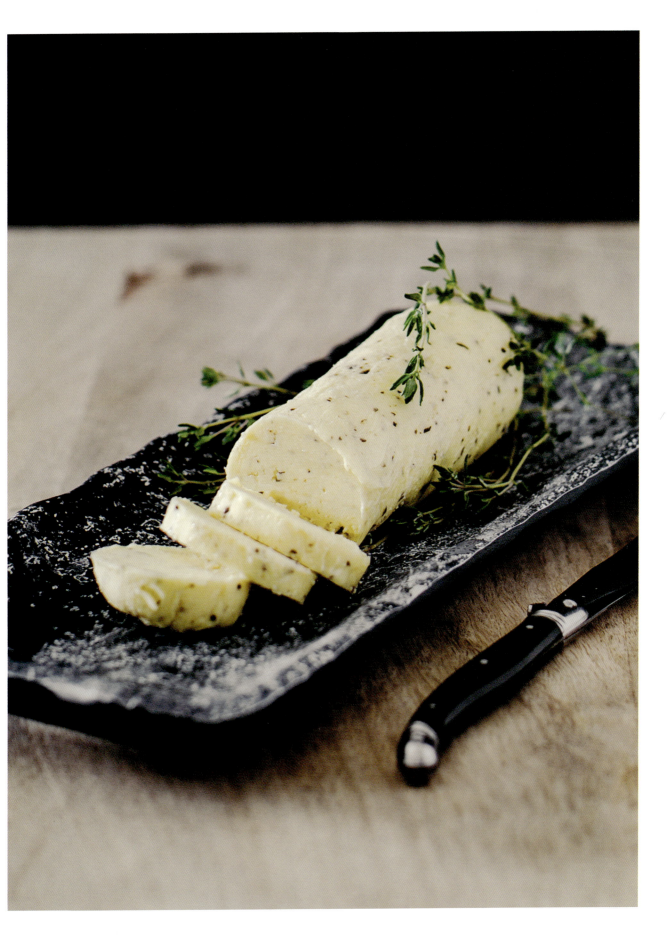

Camembert

Have you ever wondered what the difference is between camembert and brie? Basically, it's the region in France where they come from. It's also the size of the cheese, Brie is the original and is in a bigger wheel, while camembert is a small wheel. The process and ingredients are very similar.

One of the stories of how these cheeses ended up in different regions goes back to the French Revolution ... It is said that a priest who was a cheese maker in a monastery in Brie, fled the area during the French revolution. He was given shelter in a farmhouse in Normandy. As payment for his lodgings, he helped with the chores and taught the farmer's wife how to make the cheese he had been making in Brie. News soon spread and the cheese became so popular with the surrounding farmers that her daughter set up shop in the nearby village of Camembert. One day, Napoleon I was in town and tried the cheese and commented that he did love a 'good Camembert'. Hence, the cheese was named.

There are over 400 types of cheese known in France, many of them differ only by the breed of animal, the region and pasture that the dairy herd are grazing on.

Camembert

Makes 5 x 100 g (3½ oz) pieces

4 litres (135 fl oz/16 cups) non-homogenised milk
1 pinch spoon type M type starter
2 drop spoons white mould spore
1.2 ml (0.04 fl oz) liquid vegetarian rennet
20 ml (½ fl oz) boiled water, cooled
100 g (3½ oz) non-iodised salt

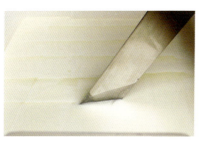

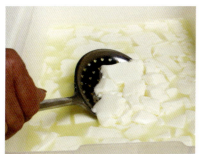

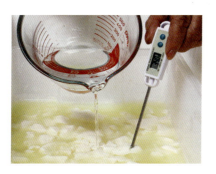

Day 1

In a large saucepan, heat the milk to 32°C (89°F). Once warmed, transfer the milk into your cheese vat. To your milk, add the type M starter and one drop spoon of white mould spore and mix in well. Leave for 1.5 hours.

Mix the liquid vegetarian rennet with the cold, pre-boiled water. Pour the diluted rennet immediately into the milk, taking care to pour it over as much of the surface as possible. Mix in well and allow the milk to set into a curd. This will take 40 minutes. Boil the jug, as you will need water at 60°C (140°F) to cook the curd in a later step.

Cut the curd

To check the curd, place the blade of a knife into the curd and lift at a 45-degree angle, looking for a clean break. If the curd parts well, it is ready to cut. Cut the curd in 3cm (1¼ inch) intervals using a curd cutting knife. Cut from top to bottom and left to right. Next, using a curd cutting rack, cut through horizontally. Allow the curd to rest for 5 minutes.

Turn the curd

Using a curd turning spoon, slide the spoon down the side of the vat and underneath the curd. Then gently lift and jiggle, bringing the curd turning spoon to the surface. Continue until all of the curd has been turned once. Rest the curd for 10 minutes and gently turn again. Rest the curd again for a further 10 minutes, then turn again. The curd will need to be turned three times total.

Cooking the curd

Using a curd turning spoon and a plastic jug, place the curd turning spoon over the mouth of the jug and press into the curd gently to drain off 1 litre (35 fl oz/4 cups) whey and replace it with 1 litre (35 fl oz/4 cups) water from the previously boiled jug. If the curd is at 30°C (86°F) the temperature of your water should be at 60°C (140°F).

Add the water slowly, bringing the temperature of the curd up to 34°C (93.2°F), maximum of 35°C (95°F). Make sure the temperature of the curd is even throughout the vat. Allow the curd to rest for 10 minutes.

Draining the whey
Taking a curd turning spoon and a plastic jug again, drain off as much of the whey as possible using the previous method. Then using a curd turning spoon ladle the curd into small camembert cheese hoops, filling to the top. Once filled, the hoops need to be placed onto a draining tray. Cover the hoops with cheesecloth and rest for 5 minutes. Invert the hoop by holding onto the cheesecloth and turning over. Continue to invert hoop five times over the next 3 to 4 hours and drain off any excess whey as you go. Leave the curd in the hoop overnight at room temperature. Make your brine solution ready for tomorrow morning by adding the non-iodised salt, dissolved in 600 ml (21 fl oz) boiling water in a container that will have the brine solution halfway up the cheese. Leave overnight.

Day 2
The next morning, add the remaining drop spoon of white mould spore to the brine solution and stir. Remove the cheese from the hoops and place into the cooled brine solution. Leave cheese for 30 minutes, turn over, then leave for another 30 minutes. Remove cheese from brine solution and place on draining rack for 24–48 hours at room temperature with no lid on. Turn cheese every 12 hours to make sure they dry evenly, removing any whey from the draining rack container.

Once your cheese feels clammy, not wet, place the lid on to drying rack container to create a humid environment. Store cheese between 10–15°C (50–59°F) for 8 to 10 days. The cheese needs to be turned every day. On day 4, the cheese will have started to grow a white mould on the exterior, this becomes the rind. After 8–10 days, your cheese will be covered with a bloom of white mould. Wrap your cheese in foil and store in the fridge at 4°C (39.2°F). The cheese should be ready to eat after 4 weeks from the day it was made.

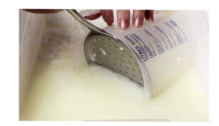
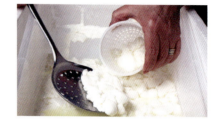
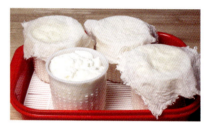
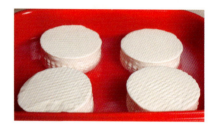
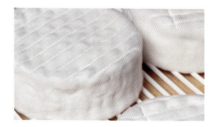
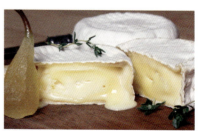

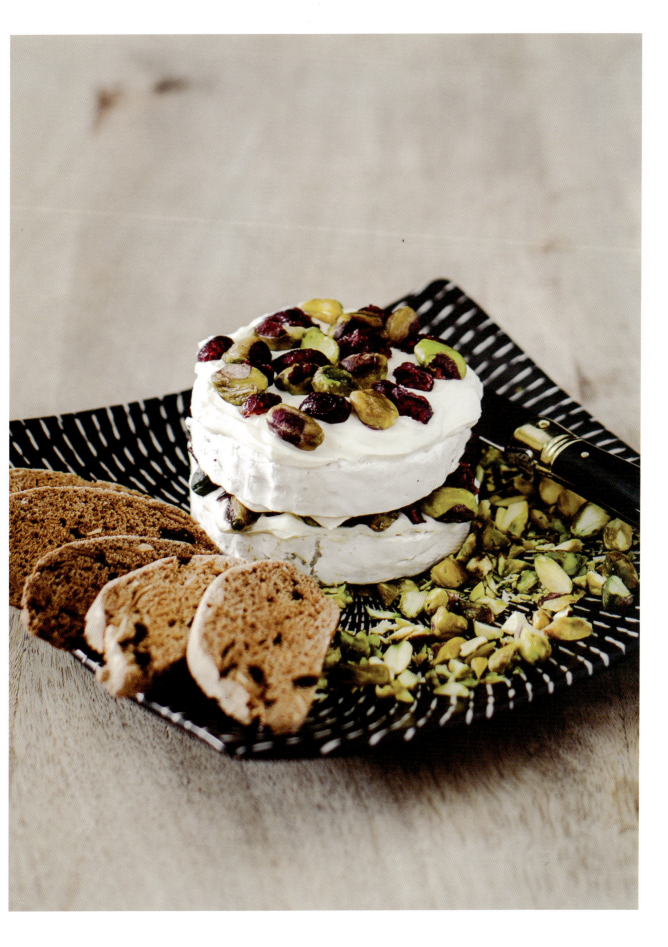

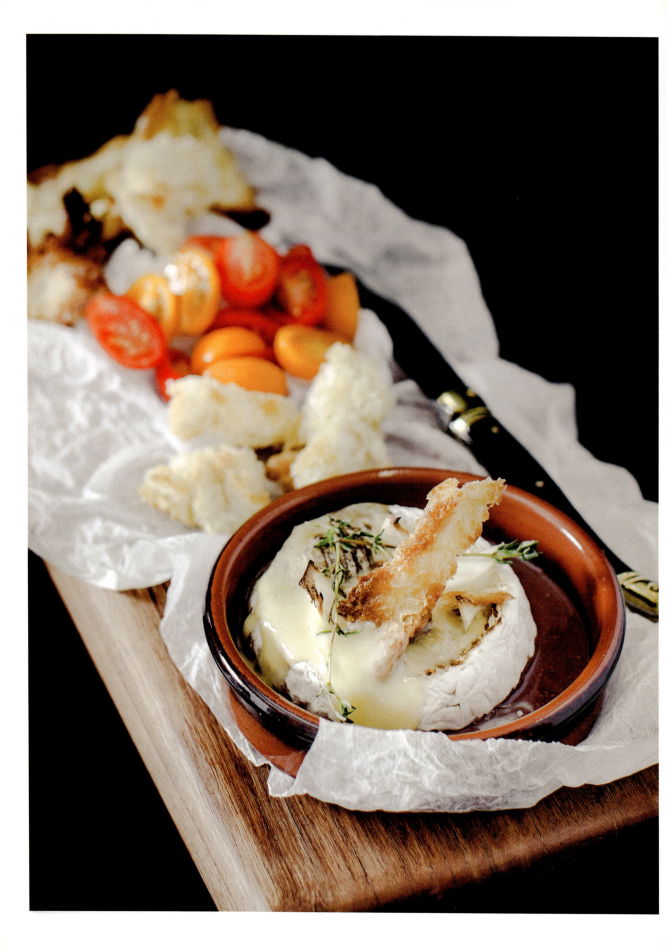

Camembert with Cranberries & Pistachios

Serves 4

1 camembert cheese
50 g (1¾ oz) mascarpone
25 g (1 oz) pistachio nuts
25 g (1 oz) dried cranberries
250 g (9 oz) biscotti, to serve

Remove the camembert from the fridge and slice in half. Spread half of the mascarpone over bottom half of the camembert.

Place half of the pistachio nuts and cranberries onto the mascarpone and top with the other half of the camembert.

Spread the remainder of the mascarpone over the camembert and sprinkle with the remaining pistachios and cranberries. Serve with biscotti.

Baked Camembert

Serves 2

1 camembert cheese
50 ml (1¾ fl oz) red wine
1 small garlic clove, finely sliced
1 thyme sprig

Unwrap a camembert and carefully slice off the top rind. Put in a small ovenproof bowl of similar size to the cheese.

Sprinkle with fresh thyme, a little finely sliced garlic and drizzle with red wine. Bake in a moderate oven until melted and serve with a baguette or ciabatta bread.

Additional ideas for baked camembert:
- Drizzle with honey, top with sliced stone fruit and crushed macadamia nuts
- Mulled wine and blueberries
- Balsamic reduction and walnuts
- Quince paste
- Champagne jelly and tarragon

Cheddar

Cheddar cheese originated in the English village of Cheddar, Somerset and is the most widely purchased and eaten cheese in the world. Cheddar is a firm, cow's milk cheese that can range in flavors from mild to sharp and in color from white to various shades of yellow and orange. A Cheddar cheese will vary from country to country, region to region and cheese maker to cheese maker.

Orange Cheddars are colored with annatto which is a natural plant extract used as a dye. Cheddars vary in flavor depending on the length of ageing and their origin. For example, Canadian Cheddars are smoother, creamier, and are known for their balance of flavor and sharpness.

As Cheddar slowly ages, it loses moisture and its texture becomes drier and crumbly. Sharpness becomes noticeable at 12 months and will increase with age. The best English Cheddar is matured for a minimum of nine months and its texture should be smooth and firm, not crumbly or rubbery.

Cheddar

Makes 900 g (2 lb)

8 litres (270 fl oz) non-homogenised milk
1 pinch spoon type M starter
2.5 ml (0.08 fl oz) liquid vegetarian rennet
2 dessertspoons non-iodised salt
20 ml (½ fl oz) boiled water, cooled

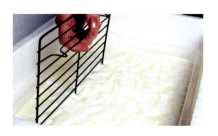

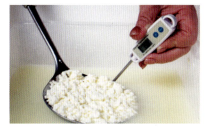

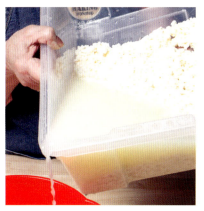

Day 1

In a large saucepan, heat the non-homogenised milk to 32°C (89°F). Once warm transfer the milk to your cheese vat. Add the type M starter to the milk. Mix the liquid vegetarian rennet with the cool, pre-boiled water. Pour the diluted rennet immediately into the milk, taking care to pour it over as much of the surface as possible. Mix in well and allow the milk to set into a curd. This will take 40 minutes.

Cut the curd

To check the curd, place the blade of a curd cutting knife into the curd and lift at a 45-degree angle, looking for a clean break. If the curd parts well, it is ready to cut. Cut the curd into 1.5 cm (⅝ inch) intervals using a curd cutting knife. Cut from top to bottom and left to right. Next, using a curd cutting rack, cut through horizontally. Allow the curd to rest for 5 minutes.

Turn the curd

Over the next hour, gently turn the curd continuously. While turning the curd, slowly cook the curd, bringing the temperature of the curd up to 39°C (102°F), do this by adding boiling water into the styrene box that the cheese vat is sitting in, making it a bain-marie. As the curd starts releasing whey this can be removed, so we are not wasting energy on heating the whey up as well as the curd. In total you will need to remove approximately 3 litres (102 fl oz/12 cups) of whey. As the curd firms up you don't need to be so gentle. Once the curd is firm and approximately the size of a grain of rice place, leave the curd to rest for 5 minutes, then drain off as much of the whey as possible.

Cheddaring the curd

Prepare the curd for cheddaring. Move the curd to one

end of the 10 litre (338 fl oz) container and leave for 30 minutes to form a slab. Cut the slab in half, and place one on top of the other half. Turn the slab of curd over every 15 minutes for 2 hours, maintaining the temperature at 38°C (100°F). Remove any whey that the curd is releasing. You may need to add more hot water into the styrene box that the cheese vat is sitting in.

Chipping the curd
This can be done by either cutting the curd with a knife into chips or by breaking the curd up with your hands. Break or cut the curd into small 1cm (½ inch) pieces.

Salting the curd
Sprinkle 1 dessertspoon of non-iodised salt into the curd and mix well. Taste the curd, if it needs more salt, add more. Transfer the salted curd into an extra large cheese hoop that is lined with cheesecloth, fold the cloth neatly over the curd and place another extra large cheese hoop on top. Press with approximately 8 kg (17 lb 10 oz) weight for 30 minutes. Remove from the press, then turn the cheese over and rearrange the cheesecloth to minimise creases. Place it back in the hoop with the other hoop on top. Press again overnight with approximately 20 kg (44 lb) weight (Some heavy cookbooks will usually do the trick).

Day 2
Remove the cheese from the hoop and cheesecloth and leave it on a draining rack to air dry for 24 to 48 hours.

Day 4
When your cheese is feeling dry, it is ready to wax. Heat your cheese wax in an old but clean saucepan until just melted. Dip the cheese into the melted wax, making sure it is well covered, usually about three layers of wax is needed to totally seal the cheese. Store your cheese at between 10–15°C (50–59°F) for eight to twelve months, turning it once a week.

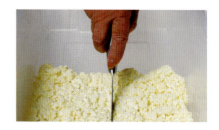
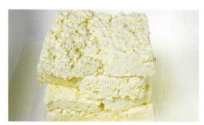
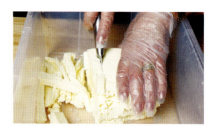
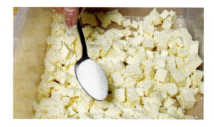
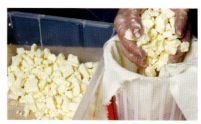
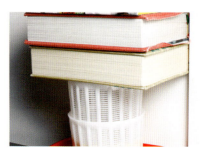

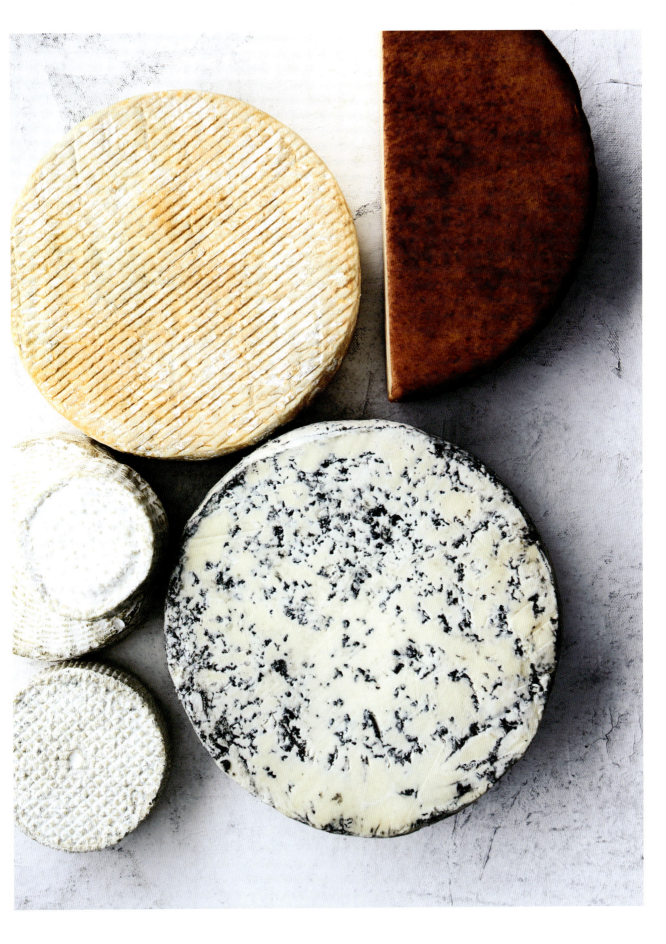

Cheddar Washed Curd

Makes 900 g (1 lb 98 oz)
A washed curd cheddar is ready to eat sooner as the washing of the curd removes lactic acid which shortens the maturation time. Being a home cheese maker, you don't want to wait twelve months, only to try the cheese and realise you forgot to add the salt!

8 litres (270 fl oz) non-homogenised milk
1 pinch spoon type M starter
2.5 ml (0.08 fl oz) liquid vegetarian rennet
2 dessertspoons of non-iodised salt
20 ml (½ fl oz) boiled water, cooled

Day 1
In a large saucepan heat the non-homogenised milk to 32°C (89°F). Once warm transfer the milk into your cheese vat. Add the type M starter to the milk. Mix the liquid vegetarian rennet with the cool, pre-boiled water. Pour the diluted rennet immediately into the milk, taking care to pour it over as much of the surface as possible. Mix in well and allow the milk to set into a curd. This will take 40 minutes.

Cut the curd
To check the curd, place the blade of a curd cutting knife into the curd and lift at a 45-degree angle, looking for a clean break. If the curd parts well, it is ready to cut. Cut the curd into 1.5 cm (⅝ inch) intervals using a curd cutting knife. Cut from top to bottom and left to right. Next, using a curd cutting rack, cut through horizontally. Allow the curd to rest for 5 minutes.

Turn the curd
Over the next hour, gently turn the curd continuously. While turning the curd, slowly cook the curd, bringing the temperature of the curd up to 39°C (102°F). Do this by adding boiling water into the outer container making it a bain-marie. As the curd starts releasing whey this can be removed, so we are not wasting energy on heating the whey up as well as the curd. In total you will need to remove approximately 3 litres (102 fl oz) whey. As the curd firms up you don't need to be so gentle. Once the curd is firm and approximately the size of a grain of rice, place 3 litres (102 fl oz/12 cups) cold water into the curd, bringing the temperature of the curd down to 30°C

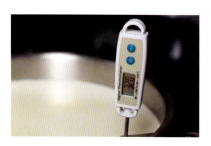
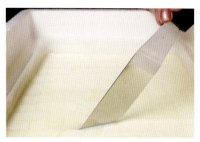
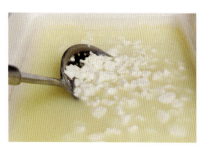

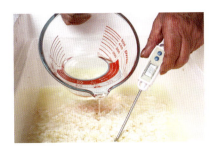
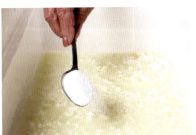
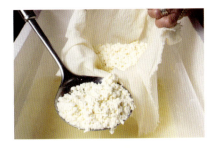
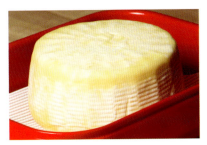
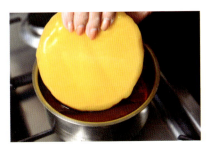

(86°F), stir for 5 minutes. Leave the curd to rest for 5 minutes, then drain off as much of the whey as possible. Sprinkle 1 dessertspoon of non-iodised salt into the curd and mix well. Taste the curd if it needs more salt add more.

Hoop the curd

Transfer the salted curd into an extra large cheese hoop that is lined with cheesecloth. Fold the cloth neatly over the curd and place another extra large cheese hoop on top. Press with approximately 8 kg (17 lb 10 oz) weight for 30 minutes. Remove from the press then turn the cheese over and rearrange the cheesecloth to minimise creases. Place it back in the hoop with the other hoop on top. Press again overnight with approximately 10 kg (22 lb) weight (Some heavy cookbooks will usually do the trick).

Day 2

Remove the cheese from the hoop and cheesecloth and leave it on a draining rack to air dry for 24 to 48 hours.

Day 4

When your cheese is feeling dry it is ready to wax. Heat your cheese wax in an old but clean saucepan until just melted. Dip the cheese into the melted wax making sure it is well covered, usually about three layers of wax is needed to totally seal the cheese. Store your cheese at between 10–15°C (50–59°F) for 8 weeks, turning it once a week.

Note

Making club cheddar is a great way to use all the little bits of leftover cheese such as cheddar, havarti, edam ... Be sure to only use semi-hard cheeses. Blend your mixture of cheeses together in a food processor, then fold through dried chilli, peppercorns or caraway seeds then re-press the cheese using a weight of approximately 8–10 kg (17–22 lb). Cryovac the cheese and store in the fridge for 2 weeks for the flavors to infuse before serving.

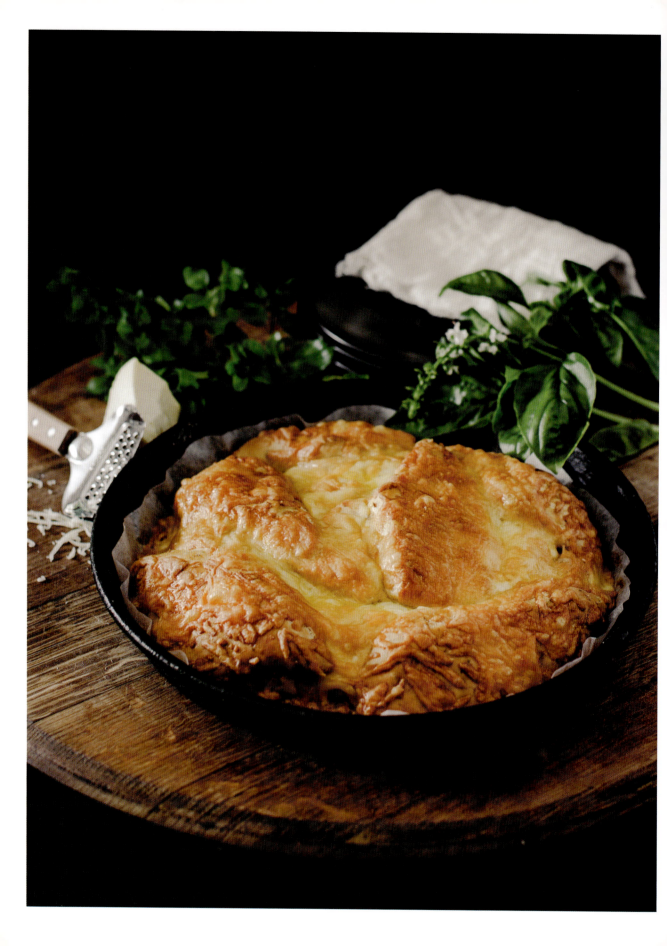

Pull-apart Bread

Serves 4

250 g (9 oz) baker's flour
1 teaspoon salt
1 teaspoon bread improver
1 teaspoon sugar
2 teaspoons dried yeast
2 teaspoons dried herbs
20 ml (½ fl oz) oil
150 ml (5 fl oz) warm water
　or whey
250 g (9 oz) grated cheddar cheese
1 egg, beaten

Combine the flour, salt, bread improver, sugar, yeast, herbs and oil. Add most of the water to bring the dough together and knead for 10 minutes until dough is smooth. (Hold back a little water to adjust moisture level as needed.)

After kneading your dough for 10 minutes, take a bit of the dough and stretch to make a window, this will tell you if the dough is ready. Allow to prove by keeping your dough covered and in a warm place. This will take approximately 1 hour.

Knock back the dough and roll out to approximately 1cm (½ inch) thick and cut into random shapes. In a lined greased round baking dish, place a third of the cut dough shapes, starting from the centre overlapping slightly to form your first layer. Don't go to the edges, as you will need room for the dough to rise and expand. Sprinkle with a third of the cheese. Place a second layer of the dough on top and sprinkle with a third of the cheese. Place the remaining dough over the first two layers.

Glaze the top layer with a beaten egg before adding the last of the cheese. Allow to prove, this will take approximately 45 minutes.

Bake at 180°C (350°F/Gas 4) for approximately 20 minutes, or until your bread is golden and sounds hollow when tapped. Your bread is best served warm.

Cheese Curds

Fresh cheese curds originated in Quebec, Canada in the 1960 as a way of utilising the surplus milk from local dairies. The squeak of the fresh cheese curds is popular as a snack, finger food, entrée or used in the comforting dish poutine.

Poutine is very simple to make it is hot potato chips or wedges served with gravy and topped with fresh curds, not the most elegant of dishes but delicious on a freezing winters day. To make the best poutine add the cheese curds at the last moment so that when you take your first bite the curds aren't melted. They are still fresh and squeaky. The hot chips or wedges need to have a bit of crunch, not soggy and of course, a good gravy.

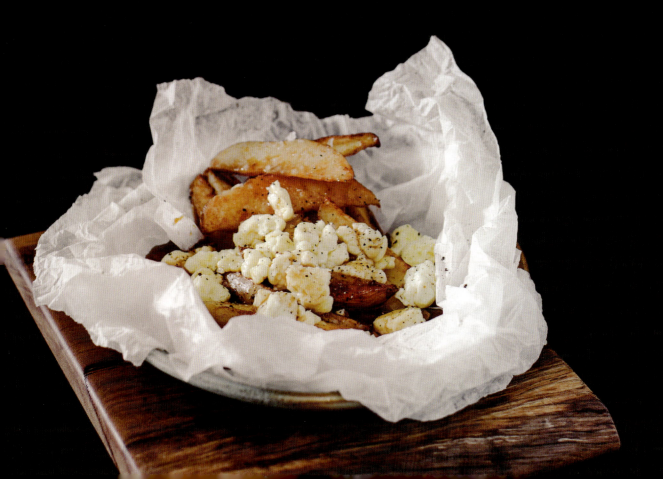

Curds

Makes 400 g (14 oz)

A French-Canadian classic. Fresh cheese curds should be eaten at room temperature; refrigeration removes the customary squeak, which is a mark of the freshness of the curd. The curds are lightly salted which makes them a moreish snack to have with a cheeky little beverage.

2 litres (70 fl oz/8 cups) un-homogenised milk
1 pinch spoon type T starter
0.5 ml (0.02 fl oz) liquid vegetarian rennet
10 ml (¼ fl oz) boiled water, cooled
20 g (¾ oz) non-iodised salt

In a saucepan, heat the un-homogenised milk to 32°C (89.6°F). Remove from heat. Add a pinch spoon of type T starter. Then mix the liquid vegetarian rennet with the cooled pre-boiled water and pour the diluted rennet mixture immediately into the milk, taking care to pour it over as much of the surface as possible. Mix in well and allow the milk to set into a curd. This will take 40 minutes.

Keep the saucepan of milk at 32°C (89.6°F) by placing the lid on the saucepan and wrapping in a clean towel. To check the curd, place the blade of a knife into the curd and lift, looking for a clean break. If the curd parts well, it is ready to cut. Cut the curd with a curd-cutting knife into 1.5–2 cm (⅝–¾ inch) cubes and rest for 5 minutes.

Place the pot on the stovetop over low heat, turning the stove on and off at regular intervals. Gently turn the curd while gradually bringing the temperature of the curd up to 40°C (104°F), this will take 10–15 minutes done correctly.

Allow the curd to rest and settle to the bottom of the pot for 30–45 minutes. Place a colander over a jug or other saucepan and pour the curds and whey into the colander to separate the curds from the whey. Keep the whey you will need this at a later step. Leave the curd to sit in the colander for approximately 1 hour to cool, then break into walnut-sized pieces. Bring the whey to boiling point add the salt and stir to dissolve, place the walnut-sized pieces of curd into the hot whey and remove from the heat.

Leave the curd in the hot whey for 1 hour, then pour through a colander. Your fresh cheese curds are ready to use! Why not try making the French-Canadian classic, Poutine? It's an easy winter warmer. Start with homemade hot chips, your cheese curds and then cover with homemade gravy. Delish!

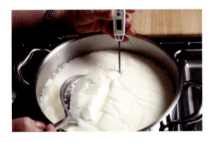
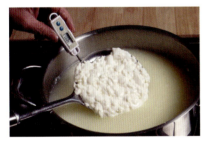
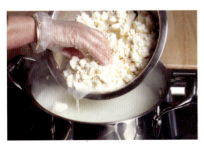

Edam

Edam is named after the town of the same name in The Netherlands. It's a semi-hard cheese that, when eaten young, has a mild and sweet flavor which changes to a slightly firmer, salty or nutty cheese with age. The Dutch took this cheese on their exploratory voyages, which gave the cheese great exposure, and its popularity spread all over the world.

Edam is always a welcomed treat that's served young with summer fruits. When aged, serve with beer, red wine and/or crusty bread.

Edam

Makes 800g (1 lb 12 oz)

8 litres (270 fl oz) non-homogenised milk
1 pinch spoon of type M starter
2.5 ml (0.08 fl oz) liquid vegetarian rennet
200 g (7 oz) non-iodised salt
25 ml (1 fl oz) boiled water, cooled

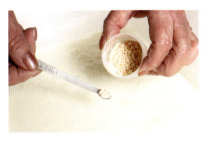

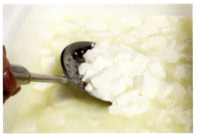

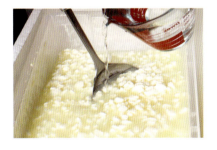

Day 1

In a large saucepan heat the non-homogenised milk to 32°C (89°F). Once warm transfer the milk into your cheese vat. Add the type M starter to the milk. Mix the liquid vegetarian rennet with the cool, pre-boiled water. Pour the diluted rennet immediately into the milk, taking care to pour it over as much of the surface as possible. Mix in well and allow the milk to set into a curd. This will take 40 minutes.

Cut the curd

To check the curd, place the blade of a curd cutting knife into the curd and lift at a 45-degree angle, looking for a clean break. If the curd parts well, it is ready to cut. Cut the curd into 1cm (½ inch) intervals using a curd cutting knife. Cut from top to bottom and left to right. Next, using a curd cutting rack, cut through horizontally. Allow the curd to rest for 5 minutes.

Turn the curd

Over the next 30 minutes, gently turn the curd, slide the spoon down the side of the vat and underneath the curd. Then gently lift and jiggle, bringing the curd turning spoon to the surface. Turn the curd gently and continuously for 30 minutes.

Remove 3 litres (102 fl oz/12 cups) whey, using a curd turning spoon and a plastic jug, place the curd turning spoon over the mouth of the jug and press into the curd. Replace the whey with 2 litres (70 fl oz/8 cups) water at 65°C (149°F) slowly add the water into the curd bringing the temperature of the curd up to 36°C (96.5°F). Continue turning the curd for another 40 minutes. Rest the curd for 10 minutes.

Drain away as much of the whey as possible. Using a curd turning spoon and a plastic jug, place the curd turning spoon over the mouth of the jug and press into the curd. Keep the whey as you will need it when pressing the curd.

Hoop the curd

Transfer the curd into an extra large cheese hoop that is lined with cheesecloth. Fold the cloth neatly over the curd and place another extra large cheese hoop on top. The hoop needs to then be placed in a saucepan or similar vessel that will hold the hoop and the kept whey. You need to press the curd under the whey, with approximately 8 kg (17 lb 10 oz) weight for 30 minutes.

Remove from the press and whey, turn the cheese over and rearrange the cheesecloth to minimise creases, then place it back in the hoop on a draining rack with the other hoop on top. Press again overnight with approximately 10 kg (22 lb) weight. (Some heavy cookbooks will usually do the trick.)

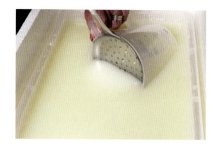

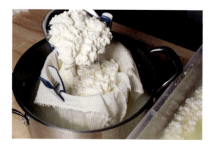

Day 2

Remove the cheese from the hoop and cheesecloth and place into a cooled brine solution. To make the brine solution mix the 200 g (7 oz) salt with 1 litre (35 fl oz/4 cups) cooled pre-boiled water. Leave the cheese for 1 hour, then turn over and leave for another hour. Remove the cheese from the brine solution and place on a draining rack for 24 hours to 48 hours at room temperature with no lid on. Turn cheese every 12 hours to make sure they dry evenly, removing any whey from the draining rack container.

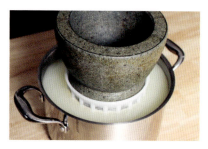

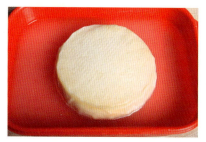

Day 4

When your cheese is feeling dry it is ready to wax. Heat your cheese wax in an old but clean saucepan until just melted. Dip the cheese into the melted wax making sure it is well covered, usually about three layers of wax is needed to totally seal the cheese. Store your cheese at between 10–15°C (50–59°F) for two to six months, turning it once a week.

Your cheese is then ready to eat! Enjoy.

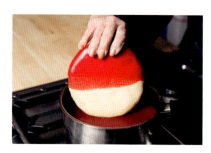

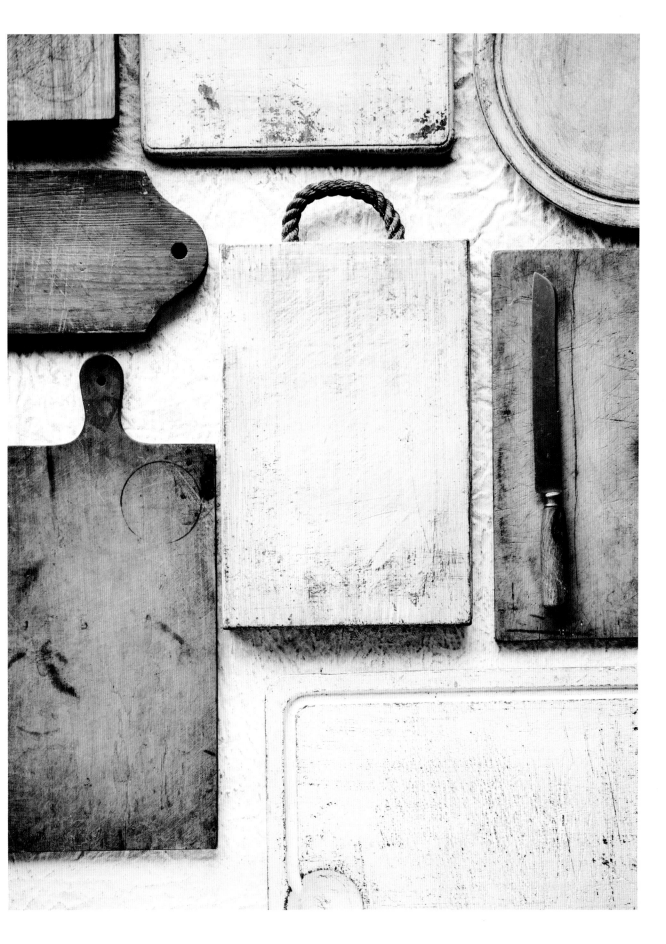

Fetta

Fetta is said to have originated in the arid hills behind Athens, where the shepherds made the cheese from ewe and goat's milk. Our fetta recipe is made using cow's milk. (There is a goat's milk fetta recipe in the goat's cheese chapter on page 148).

Fetta is a brined cheese and is ready to eat only four to five days after making. This is one of the easiest cheeses to make and if they could produce it in the arid hills of Athens, surely you can make it in your kitchen.

Fetta

Makes 2 x 350 g (12½ oz) pieces

4 litres (135 fl oz/16 cups) non-homogenised milk
1 pinch of type M starter
1 drop of Lipase powder
1 ml (0.03 fl oz) liquid vegetarian rennet
40 ml (1¼ fl oz) boiled water, cooled
120 g (4¼ oz) non-iodised salt

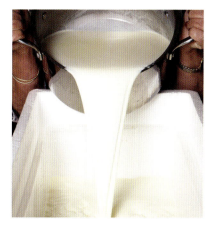

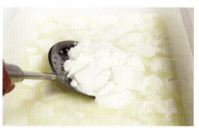

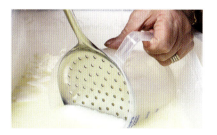

Day 1

In a large saucepan, heat the non-homogenised milk to 32°C (89°F). Once warmed, transfer the milk into your cheese vat. Add the type M starter to the milk. Stir. Add the lipase to 20 ml (½ fl oz) cooled pre-boiled water, stir and pour into the warm milk. Mix thoroughly.

Mix the liquid vegetarian rennet with 20 ml (½ fl oz) cooled, pre-boiled water. Pour the diluted rennet immediately into the milk, taking care to pour it over as much of the surface as possible. Mix in well. Leave the milk to rest for 60 to 90 minutes and the milk will set into a curd.

Cut the curd

To check the curd, place the blade of a knife into the curd and lift at a 45-degree angle, looking for a clean break. If the curd parts well, it is ready to cut. Cut the curd in 1.5 cm (⅝ inch) intervals using a curd cutting knife. Cut from top to bottom and left to right. Next, using a curd cutting rack to cut through horizontally. Allow curd to rest for 5 minutes.

Turn the curd

Using a curd turning spoon, slide the spoon down the side of the vat and underneath the curd. Then gently lift and jiggle, bringing the curd turning spoon to the surface. Continue until all of the curd has been turned once. Rest for 1 hour and turn for the second time. Rest the curd for 1 hour then turn for the third time. Rest the curd for 10 minutes. The curd needs to be turned a total of three times.

Draining the whey

Using a curd turning spoon and a plastic jug, place the curd turning spoon over the mouth of the jug and press into the curds so the whey can seep through the spoon to gently drain off as much of the whey as possible.

If you want to add a little flavor to your fetta, before hooping the curd you can add dried herbs, dried chilli, some fennel or caraway seed.

Hooping the curd

Then, using a curd turning spoon, place the curd into the square cheese hoops, filling each hoop to the top. Do not go back and top up the cheese hoops until you have filled both hoops. (They sink down quickly.) Once filled, the hoops need to be placed onto draining trays. Cover the hoops with cheesecloth. Invert the hoops by holding onto the cheesecloth and turning each hoop over.

Continue to invert the hoops five times over the next 3–4 hours and drain off any excess whey as you go.

Leave the fetta curd in the hoops overnight at room temperature.

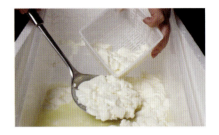

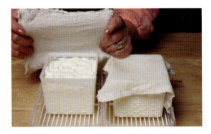

Day 2

Take the fetta out of the cheese hoops and air dry for up to two days on a draining rack at room temperature. Turn the cheese morning and night, draining off the whey each time.

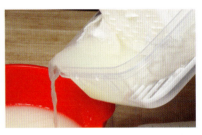

Day 3 or 4

Make up a brine solution by adding 120 g (4¼ oz) of non-iodised salt to 1 litre (35 fl oz/4 cups) of boiling water and allow to cool. Put the fetta in the cooled brine solution; make sure the brine covers the cheeses. The fetta is ready to consume after 24 hours of being in the brine. It can be stored in brine, in the fridge for 3 months if you replace the brine every 3 weeks.

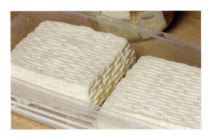

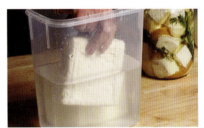

Persian Fetta

Makes 2 x 350 g (12 oz) pieces

4 litres (135 fl oz/16 cups) non-homogenised milk
1 pinch of type M starter
1 drop of lipase powder
1 ml (0.03 fl oz) liquid vegetarian rennet
40 ml (1¼ fl oz) boiled water, cooled
100 g (3½ oz) non-iodised salt

Follow the steps for fetta (p73–74) with the following adjustments:

Cut the curd into 2.5–5 cm cubes, (1–2 inches). When placing the fetta in brine, make a brine solution by mixing 100 g (3½ oz) non-iodised salt and 1 litre (35 fl oz/4 cups) of boiling water. Allow to cool. Place the fetta in the brine for 24 hours. After 24 hours, remove the fetta from the brine. Dice the fetta into cubes, place in a container and cover with a light oil that won't solidify in the fridge. We use sunflower oil. Flavor the oil, for example adding lime zest and garlic, chilli and mixed herbs.

Notes

If you like a creamy Danish fetta, try adding 160 ml (5¼ fl oz) pure cream as an addition to the milk and follow the Persian fetta recipe.

If you are wanting to marinate your fetta, this can be done after the cheese has been in the brine for 24 hours. Place your cheese in a clean sterile jar with flavors of your choice. We use a bruised garlic clove, or chilli, herbs and peppercorns are also good. Make sure the cheese is totally covered in oil. We use sunflower oil as it does not solidify.

A little bit of fetta makes life better ...

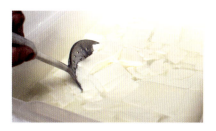

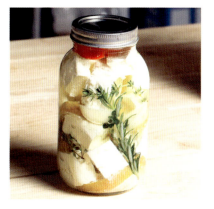

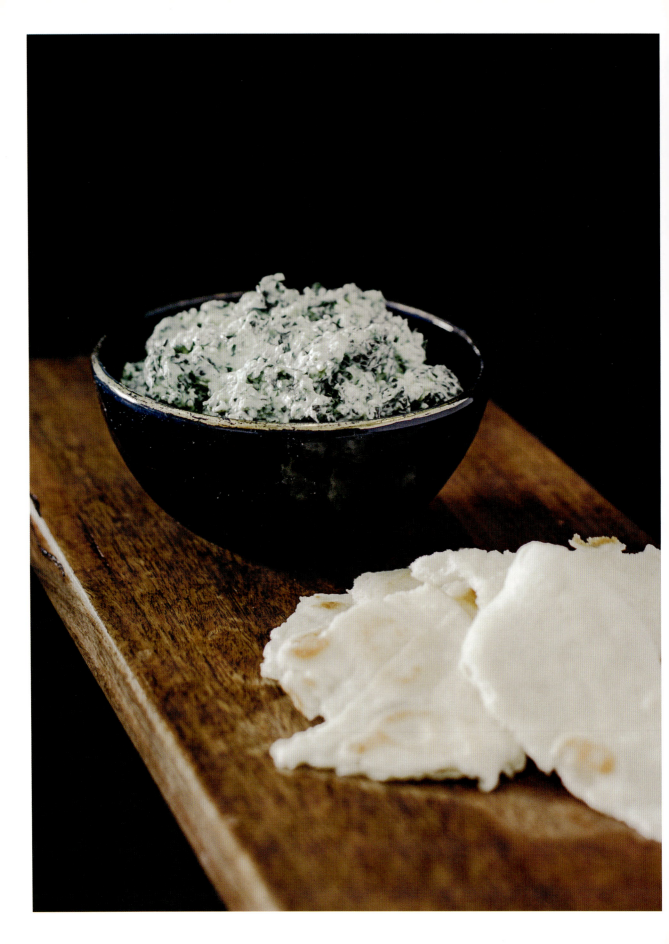

Spinach & Fetta Dip

Makes 650 g (23 oz)

250 g (9 oz) spinach, blanched, chopped
200 g (7 oz) crumbled fetta cheese
200 g (7 oz) quark
2 garlic cloves, crushed
⅛ teaspoon nutmeg

Process all of the ingredients in a food processor until blended. Season with pepper only, as fetta will be salty.

Serve with toasted fresh flat bread.

You can store this dip in an airtight container in the fridge for up to 7 days.

Fetta Tart

Serves 6

Pastry
90 g (3¼ oz) butter
120 g (4¼ oz) plain (all-purpose) flour

Cheese filling
200 g (7 oz) fetta cheese
200 g (7 oz) quark
200 g (7 oz) mascarpone
2 eggs

To make the pastry, place the butter and flour into a food processor and process until combined. Continue processing and dribble in a little water until the dough comes together. Shape into a rectangular shape and wrap in plastic wrap. Place in the fridge to rest for 30 minutes.

Preheat the oven to 180°C (350°F). Roll out the pastry to fit into a rectangle tart tin and blind bake for 15 minutes.

To make the cheese filling, process the ingredients in a food processor until smooth, then pour into the pre-cooked pastry base and bake in for 20 minutes.

Serve with semi-dried tomato, marinated mushrooms, pesto and salad.

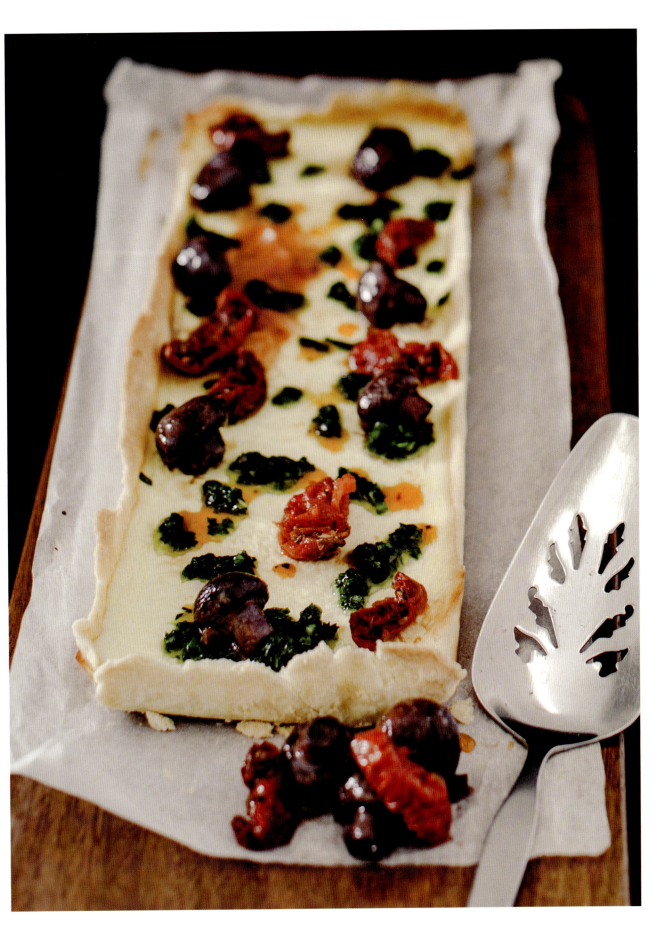

Haloumi

Haloumi originated in Cyprus, it is a quick cheese to produce and can be eaten on the same day it is made or stored in a brine solution for several weeks. Although it is traditionally made with a blend of Sheep's and Goat's milk, the Cow's milk version is still very good.

Sometimes called 'squeaky' cheese due to the feel of its texture between your teeth, it is slightly salty in flavor and is a popular cheese to cook on a grill plate or barbeque. It goes well with Mediterranean flavors and is also a hit in our breakfast dish of poached eggs, Haloumi and hollandaise sauce.

Haloumi

Makes 2 x 300 g (10½ oz) pieces

4 litres (135 fl oz/16 cups) non-homogenised milk
1 ml (0.03 fl oz) liquid vegetarian rennet
20 ml (½ fl oz) boiled water, cooled
60 g (2¼ oz) non-iodised salt

Pour the milk into a large saucepan and heat the milk to 32°C (89°F). Remove from the heat. Add the liquid vegetarian rennet to the cooled, boiled water. Pour the diluted rennet over the surface of the milk and stir thoroughly. Keep the saucepan of milk at 32°C (89°F) by placing the lid on the saucepan and wrapping in a clean towel. Leave the milk to set into a curd. This will take 40 minutes.

Cut the curd
To check the curd, place the blade of a knife into the curd and lift at a 45-degree angle, looking for a clean break. If the curd parts well, it is ready to cut. Cut the curd with a curd-cutting knife into 1.5–2 cm (⅝–1 inch) cubes and rest for 5 minutes.

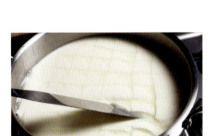

Turn and cook the curd
Place the pot back on the stovetop over low heat, turning the stove on and off at regular intervals. Gently turn the curd while gradually bringing the temperature of the curd up to 40°C (104°F), this will take 10–15 minutes when done correctly. The curd should change in appearance from a silken tofu to a scramble egg like consistency.

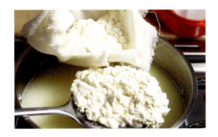

Hooping the curd
Allow the curd to rest and settle to the bottom of the pot for 30–45 minutes. Using a curd turning spoon, lift the curd out of the saucepan and place the curds equally into two square hoops, lined with cheesecloth. Keep the whey, you will need this at a later step. Fold the cloth neatly over the curd and stack another square hoop on top. Press with at least 4 kg (8 lb 13 oz) for 30 minutes. Unwrap the cheese, turn the cheese over and neatly fold back into the cheesecloth. Repress the cheese for another 1.5 hours with 4 kg (8 lb 13 oz) of weight (a couple of heavy cook books usually do the trick).

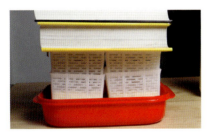

After the cheese has been pressed, bring the whey to boiling point and remove from the heat. Unwrap the cheese and place in the hot whey for 1 hour. Remove the cheese from the hot whey after 1 hour and place on a draining rack in the fridge overnight. Prepare a brine bath by mixing 60 g (2¼ oz) non-iodised salt to 500 ml (17 fl oz/2 cups) boiling water and set aside to cool. Once the brine solution has cooled, add the haloumi into the cool brine.

Note

Haloumi can be consumed after 24 hours in the brine bath or stored in the fridge for up to 2 months in the brine. Be sure to change the brine bath every 3 weeks to keep your haloumi fresh.

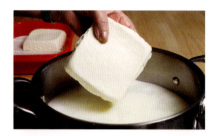

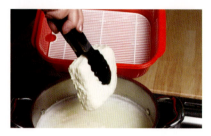

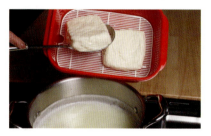

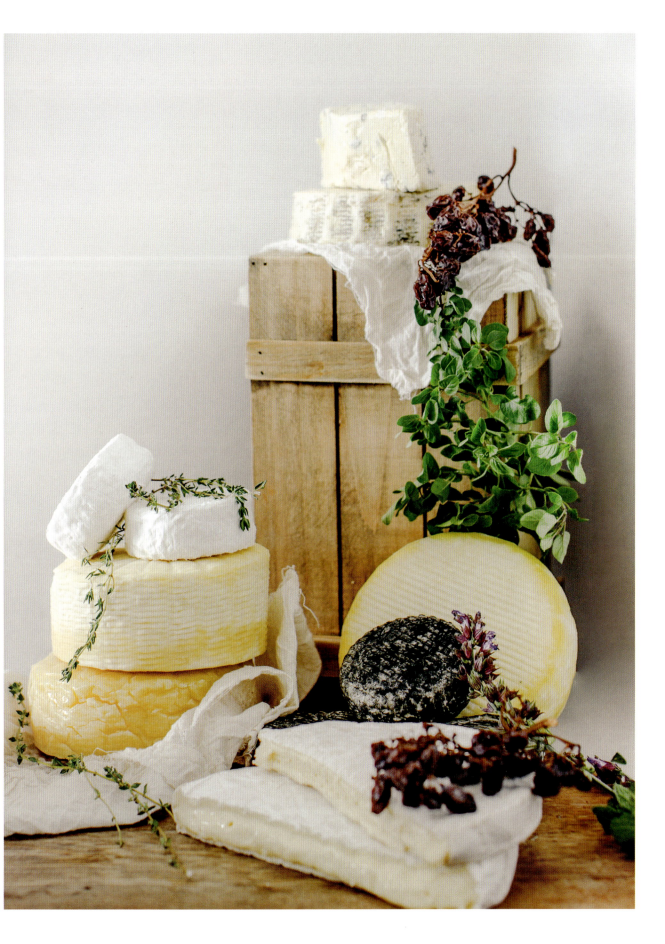

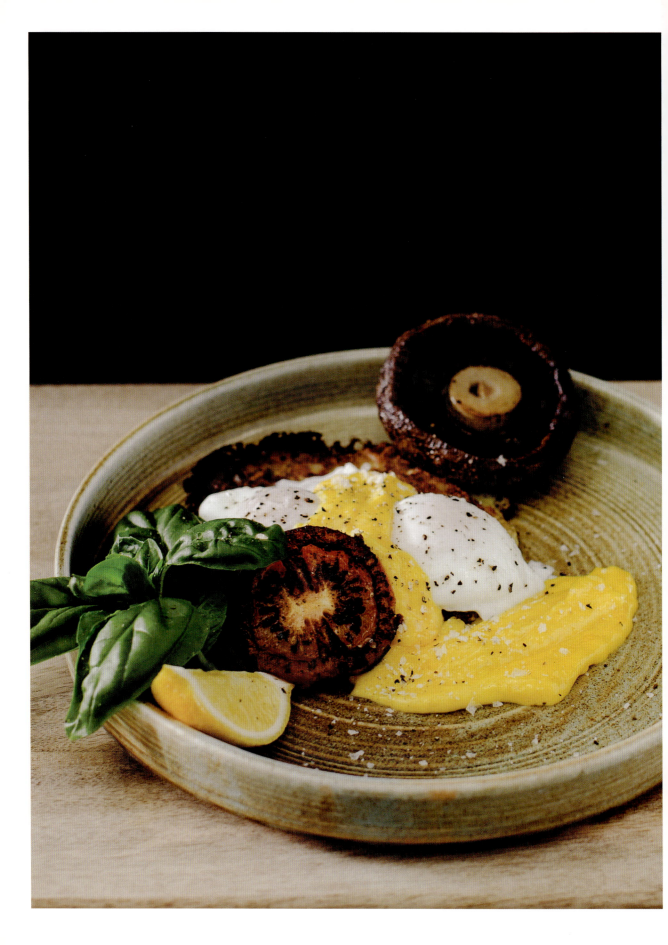

Haloumi Hash with Eggs Benedict

Serves 6

Haloumi Hash
400 g (14 oz) désirée potatoes
300 g (10½ oz) homemade haloumi cheese
1 tablespoon plain (all-purpose) flour
1 egg

Hollandaise Sauce
5 eggs
500 g (1 lb 2 oz) clarified butter
30 ml (1 fl oz) white vinegar
30 ml (1 fl oz) water
white pepper, to season

12 eggs
3 tomatoes
6 portobello mushrooms
oil, for pan-frying
pinch of white pepper and salt
squeeze of lemon or lime juice
lemon or lime wedge, to serve
basil leaves, to garnish

To make the haloumi hash, grate the potato into the bowl. Using your hands, squeeze out the excess moisture. Grate the haloumi. Add the haloumi to the grated potato, then mix in the flour and egg. Divide into six portions and set aside.

To make the hollandaise sauce, place the vinegar, water and pepper into a saucepan and slowly bring to the boil, reducing by two-thirds. Pour into a mixing bowl and allow to cool. Add the egg yolks. Using a fine whisk, beat the mixture over a warm to hot water bath until the mixture is light, with the consistency of thin cream. Remove from the heat and continue whisking until the mixture cools. Melt the butter until it splits or clarifies. Add the clarified butter slowly while continuously whisking the mixture until it thickens. Season with salt and a little lemon juice. The sauce will keep for a couple of hours if kept between 30–37°C (86–98.6°F).

Preheat the oven to 180°C (350°F). Cut the tomatoes in half and place on a baking tray. Roast in the oven until they just start to break down.

Heat the oil in a frying pan heat until hot. Pan-fry the portobello mushrooms and the haloumi hash browns until golden, then place in the oven to keep warm until you are ready to serve.

Poach the eggs until soft boiled, serve 2 eggs per person.

To plate up, place the haloumi hash on the plate, top with 2 poached eggs and the oven-roasted tomato. Place the portobello mushrooms to the side, top the dish with the hollandaise and garnish with a wedge of lemon or lime and fresh basil leaves.

Note
You will need 18 eggs in total for this recipe: 12 for poaching, 5 for the hollandaise sauce and 1 for the haloumi hash.

Greek Baked Cheese

Serves 4 as a side as a Tapas dish

Melbourne has the largest Greek population outside of Greece and I love Greek food! So on a mission we went to find a traditional Greek restaurant selling home style Greek food in Melbourne. We found it. Tsindos Greek Restaurant in the Greek precinct in Melbourne and this is my take on one of the delicious dishes we had, Greek Baked Cheese.

100 g (3½ oz) haloumi cheese
100 g (3½ oz) fetta cheese
15 cherry tomatoes
2 small red chilli
2 garlic clove, finely sliced
6 thyme sprigs
2 oregano sprigs

Crumble the homemade haloumi and fetta into a small flat baking dish, making sure the base of the dish is covered with the cheeses.

Halve the cherry tomatoes and scatter evenly over the top of the cheese.

Remove the seeds from the chilli and finely chop them. Scatter over the cheese.

Place the sliced garlic and the thyme on top of the cheese and tomato. Remove the oregano leaves from the stalks and scatter over the top. Preheat the oven to 180°C (350°F).

Once assembled, bake for approximately 10 minutes, or until the cheese is melted.

Serve with crusty bread, smashed potato or lightly cooked greens of your choice.

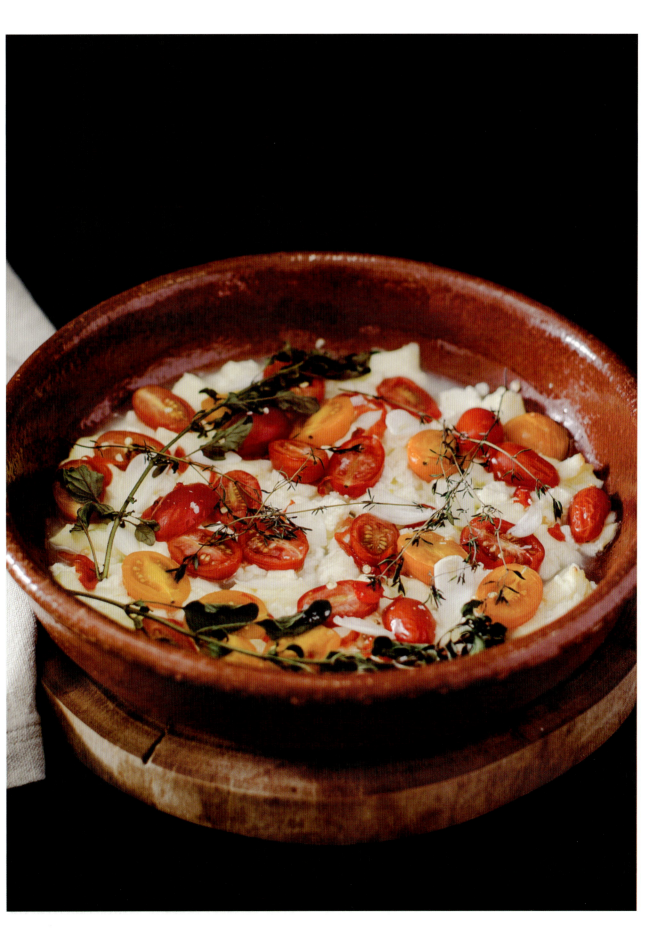

Havarti

Havarti is Denmark's most famous cheese. It has a deliciously mild buttery, rich flavor and its soft texture makes it a perfect accompaniment on any cheese platter. Havarti also melts well and makes a lovely addition to mac and cheese or a cheese toasty. We find this semi hard cheese is best eaten young. Although it can be stored for up to 6 months the flavor will change from mild to sharp depending on its age. The cheese is waxed to keep airtight and moisture retained. This ensures the cheese is always smooth and delicious. We also cryovac it in order to store it for 6 months.

Havarti

Makes 6 x 175g (6 oz) pieces

8 litres (270 fl oz) non-homogenised milk
1 pinch of type M starter
2.5 ml (0.08 fl oz) liquid vegetarian rennet
25 ml (1 fl oz) boiled water, cooled
200 g (7 oz) non-iodised salt
2 litres (70 fl oz/8 cups) water, chilled

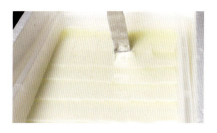

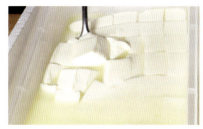

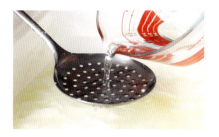

Day 1

In a large saucepan, heat the un-homogenised milk to 33°C (91°F). Once warm, transfer the milk to your cheese vat. Add the type M starter to the milk. Mix the vegetarian rennet with the cooled, pre-boiled water. Pour the rennet immediately into the milk, taking care to pour it over as much of the surface as possible. Mix in well and allow the milk to set into a curd. This will take 40 minutes.

Cut the curd

To check the curd, place the blade of a curd cutting knife into the curd and lift at a 45-degree angle, looking for a clean break. If the curd parts well, it is ready to cut. Cut the curd into 2.5 cm (1 inch) intervals using a curd cutting knife. Cut from top to bottom and left to right. Next, using a curd cutting rack, cut through horizontally. Allow the curd to rest for 5 minutes.

Turn the curd

Over the next 20 minutes, gently start to turn the curd. With havarti, you need to be extra gentle, so VERY gently lift and jiggling the curd. This will be enough movement to start encouraging the whey to be released.

Draining the whey

Using a curd turning spoon and a plastic jug, place the curd turning spoon over the mouth of the jug and press into the curds so the whey can seep through the spoon to gently remove 2 litres (70 fl oz/8 cups) of whey.

Cooking the curd

Replace the 2 litres (70 fl oz/8 cups) of whey with 2 litres (70 fl oz/8 cups) of water at 65°C (149°F). Pour the water through your slotted spoon to distribute it evenly without upsetting the curd. Gently move the curd around, bringing the temperature of the curd up to 38° (100.4°F). Over the next hour, gently turn the curd around every 10 minutes.

Cooling the curd

Remove 4 litres (135 fl oz/16 cups) of the whey and replace with the 2 litres (67.5 fl oz) chilled water, bringing the temperature of the curd down to 28°C (82.4°F). Let the curd rest for 5 minutes, then drain off all the whey and briefly and gently turn the curd to encourage a little more whey from the curd. Place the curd into hoops and place another hoop on top. Weigh the hoop down to press with approximately 4 kg (8 lb 13 oz) for 5 minutes, then invert the curd in the hoops and press again for 5 minutes. This is all the pressing required for this cheese. Over the next 2 hours invert the hoops four times.

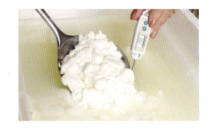
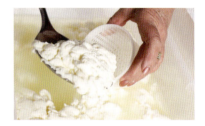
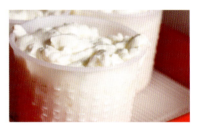

Place water into a vessel that will hold all the curd and ensure it will come halfway up the side of the curd. Place the vessel of water into the fridge to cool. After the curd has been inverted four times, remove the curd from the hoops and place into the cool water for 2 hours, 1 hour each side. Next, make a brine solution by adding 200 g (7 oz) non-iodised salt into 1 litre (35 fl oz/4 cups) boiling water. Allow enough time for this to cool. Take the curd from the cold water and place into the brine solution for 3 hours, 1.5 hours on each side. Remove the curd from the brine solution and place onto a draining rack. Dry the cheese at room temperature for 24 to 48 hours until dry.

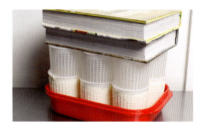

Day 2 or 3

When your cheese is feeling dry, it is ready to wax. Heat your cheese wax in an old but clean saucepan until it has just melted. Dip the cheese into the melted wax, making sure it is well covered, usually about three layers of wax is needed to totally seal the cheese. Store you cheese at between 10–15°C (50–59°F) for 6 weeks, turning once a week. Your cheese is ready to eat at 6 weeks and can be stored in a regular fridge for up to 3 months.

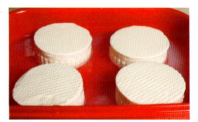

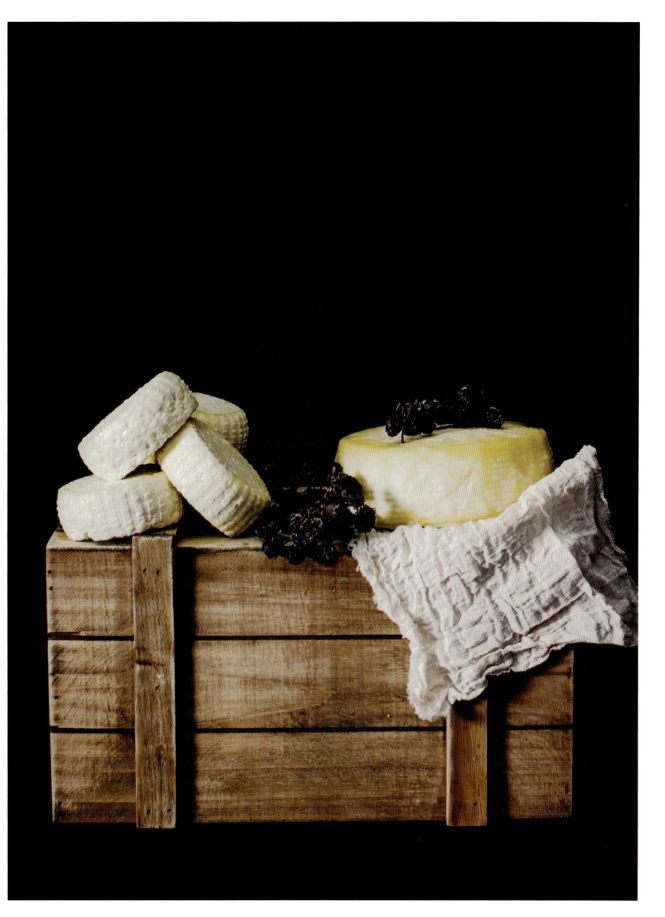

Kefir

Kefir is an ancient fermented dairy product consumed in high volumes in Russia and many Eastern European countries. Additionally, small niches have existed in Norway, Sweden, Germany and several other countries. Kefir is a cultured, enzyme rich food. Its friendly micro-organisms help balance your inner gut health and it is believed to be more nutritious and therapeutic than yoghurt. It supplies complete protein, essential minerals, as well as B vitamins.

As well as the added nutritional benefit, Kefir is thought to contain even more of those good bacteria than yoghurt, which we now know is essential to our overall heath and well being.

Both kefir and yoghurt contain beneficial bacteria but they are of different types. Yoghurt is full of beneficial bacteria that keep the digestive system clean and it provides food for the friendly bacteria that reside in our digestive track. Kefir, on the other hand, can actually colonize in the intestinal tract.

Kefir

Makes 250 g (9 oz)

1 pinch of kefir starter culture
1 litre (35 fl oz/4 cups) UHT milk

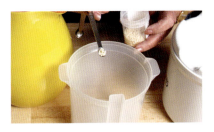

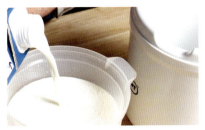

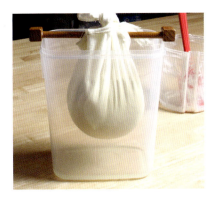

In a large container, combine the kefir starter with the UHT milk. Leave on the kitchen bench for 10 hours, or up to 36 hours. Leave it until is has set—this will depend on the temperature. Place the container in the fridge and allow to chill through completely. It is now ready to eat.

If you want your kefir thicker, once chilled, remove the lid from the container and cover with cheesecloth. Holding down the sides tightly, turn the kefir out into a colander that is lined with cheesecloth and sitting in a jug or bowl, to catch the whey. Tie opposite corners of the cheesecloth over a wooden spoon and hang over a container in the fridge for 24–48 hours. Remove from the cheesecloth and your kefir is ready for making your favorite dip!

Store your kefir in an airtight container in the fridge. Your kefir will last in the fridge for up to 1 week.

Mascarpone

Mascarpone comes from an area southwest of Milan in Italy. It was first made in the early 17th century. It is soft and buttery. Its delicate flavor and extra creamy texture makes it an absolute delight to use in either sweet or savory dishes.

This cultured cheese is sure to become a favorite in your house. I use mascarpone instead of crème fraîche or sour cream as it is beautiful to cook with. Try folding it through pasta or risotto, spread a layer in lasagne or, of course, make a tiramisu. You can also mix a little icing sugar and vanilla bean paste through it and have it with scones.

Mascarpone

Makes 500 g (1 lb 2 oz)

1 pinch of Thermophilic starter culture (type T starter)
700 ml (24 fl oz) UHT milk
300 ml (10½ fl oz) pure cream

In a yoghurt pot, combine the type T starter with the milk and cream. Mix thoroughly. Incubate in your yoghurt maker for a minimum of 16 hours. Place the yoghurt pot container in the fridge and allow to chill completely.

Remove the lid from the container and cover with cheesecloth. Holding down the sides tightly and turn out into a colander that is sitting in a jug. Tie the opposite corners of the cheesecloth over a wooden spoon and hang over a container in the fridge for 24–48 hours.

Remove from the cheesecloth and your mascarpone is ready for eating! Store your Mascarpone in an airtight container in the fridge. Your mascarpone will keep in the fridge for up to 1 week.

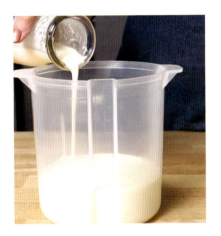

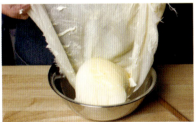

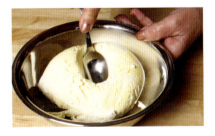

Mascarpone & White Wine Fettuccine

Serves 4

400 g (14 oz) fresh fettuccini
250 g (9 oz) mascarpone
100 ml (3½ fl oz) dry white wine
12 kalettes or broccolini
dill sprigs, to garnish
salt and pepper, to season

Bring a saucepan of water to the boil. Add the kalettes or broccolini and cook for 2 minutes (do not over cook), then remove from the boiling water and set aside.

Cook the fettuccini following the packet instructions. If using fresh pasta, cook for 3 minutes, or until *al dente*.

Meanwhile, add the mascarpone and wine into a large frying pan (it will need to be large enough to hold all the pasta). Stir over medium heat until combined and warm, do not boil.

When the pasta is cooked, add it to the mascarpone and white wine sauce and stir through. Season to taste.

To serve, divide the pasta between four pasta bowls. Place 3 kalettes or broccolini on each bowl, garnish with dill and season with salt and freshly cracked black pepper.

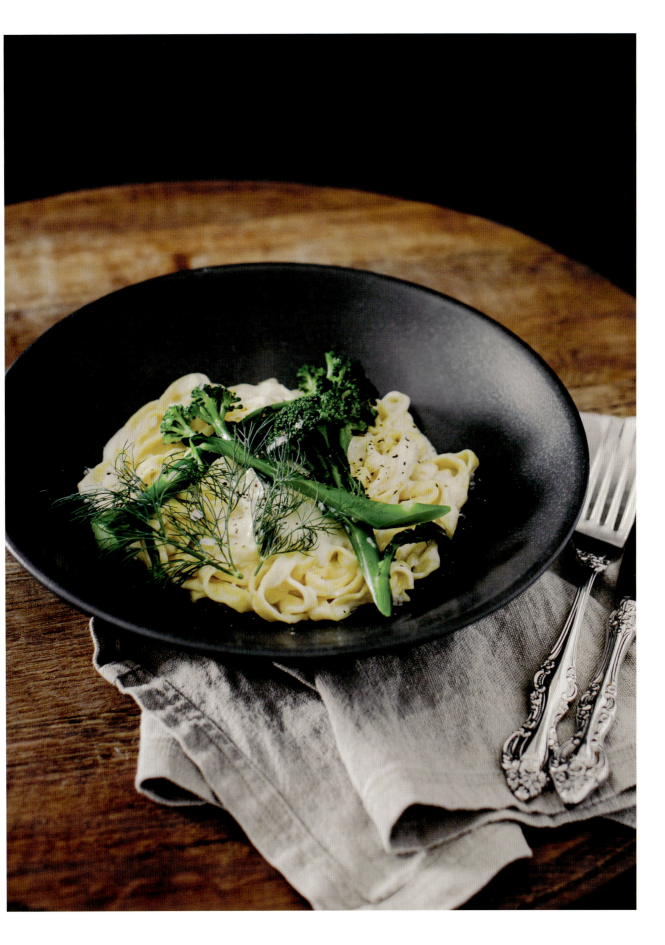

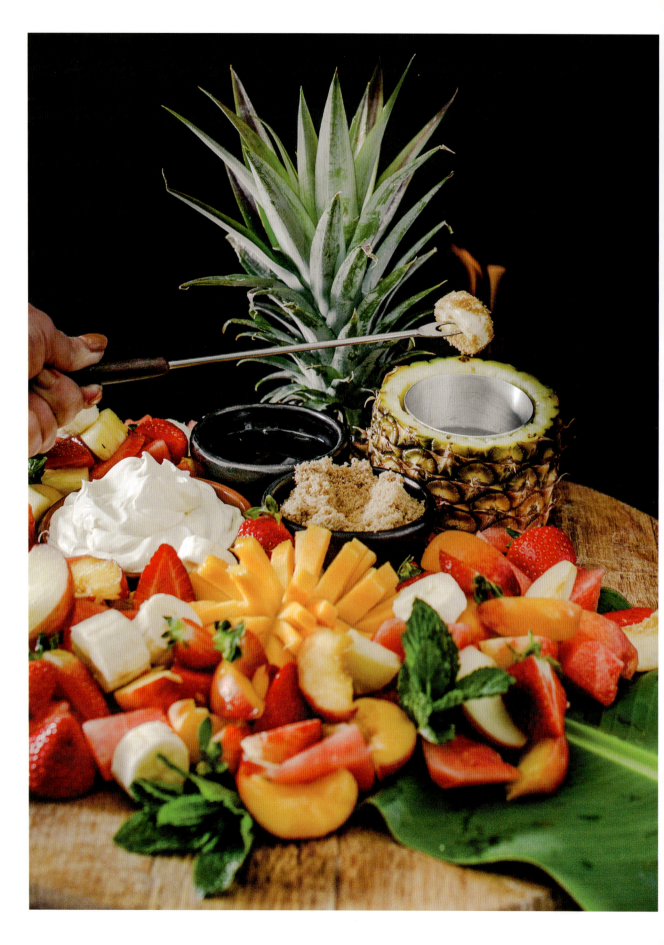

Barrenjoey

Serves 6

This has been our family's favorite summer dessert for decades. Back in the early '70s, the couple that lived in the Barrenjoey lighthouse at Palm Beach in Sydney held overnight parties for groups of people. My family went to a New Year's Eve celebration there and recall it as 'The Best Night EVER!'. They were served this for dessert and they found it to be a fantastic food sharing experience. There is nothing quite as good as fresh fruit to end a barbecue. This dish is delicious and fun. Guests spear a piece of fruit, dip it in rum, roll it in brown sugar, then hold it over a flame until the sugar caramelises. Finally, it is dipped in sweetened mascarpone.

2 pineapples, with their tops on
1 banana
1 punnet strawberries
a few pieces of whatever fruit is in season, such as stone fruit, grapes, etc.
mint leaves, to garnish
125 ml (4 fl oz/½ cup) rum
100 g (3½ oz/½ cup) brown sugar
500 g (1 lb 2 oz) sweetened mascarpone

Methylated spirits

Choose ripe pineapples with the green top on. Cut one pineapple from bottom to top, into four pieces, cutting carefully through the green top. Then cut the flesh only, don't cut through the skin. Cut into small wedges, then run a knife along the base of the pineapple under the wedges to release them form the outer shell. Set aside.

Take the other pineapple, cut off the top about a quarter of the way down using a sharp knife to hollow out the inside of the pineapple. Keep the hollowed out pineapple pieces with the pineapple wedges. Then place a flameproof small metal or ceramic ramekin into the hollowed out pineapple. This is to hold the methylated sprits that we caramelised the fruit over (we use a half of a beer can).

Place the hollowed out pineapple in the centre of a large wooden platter that is covered with a banana leaf or similar. Arrange the pineapple quarters and all the other fresh fruit around the plater. Place a small bowl with the brown sugar and another with the rum onto the platter, then fill a larger bowl with the sweetened mascarpone. When ready to serve the dessert, fill the ramekin in the pineapple three-quarters full with methylated spirits and set aflame. Dip the fruit into the rum, roll in the sugar, then caramelise over the flame. Dip into the mascarpone.

Note
If serving children, have a bowl of orange juice for them to dip in, rather than the rum!

Monterey Jack

Monterey Jack is from Monterey County in California. How it came to be goes back to the 1700s. A cheese called Queso del Pais was introduced into Southern California by Spanish missionaries. After the missionaries left, local farmers continued to make the cheese. Their method of cheesemaking eventually evolved into one of the most popular American cheeses, which is affectionately known as Jack cheese. Monterey Jack is a mild flavored cheese that melts beautifully, making it ideal for cooking and a great addition to Mexican dishes.

Monterey Jack

Makes 900 g (2 lb)

8 litres (270 fl oz) non-homogenised milk
1 pinch spoon of type M starter
2.5 ml (0.08 fl oz) liquid vegetarian rennet
120 g (4¼ oz) non-iodised salt
20 ml (½ fl oz) boiled water, cooled

Place 6 litres (204 fl oz) of water in the fridge as you will need it later

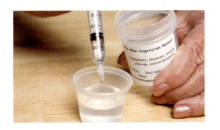

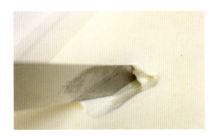

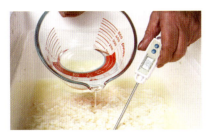

Day 1
In a large saucepan, heat the non-homogenised milk to 30°C (86°F). Once warm, transfer the milk into your cheese vat. Add the type M starter to the milk. Mix the liquid vegetarian rennet with the cool, pre-boiled water. Pour the diluted rennet immediately into the milk, taking care to pour it over as much of the surface as possible. Mix in well and allow the milk to set into a curd. This will take 1 hour.

Cut the curd
To check the curd, place the blade of a curd cutting knife into the curd and lift at a 45-degree angle, looking for a clean break. If the curd parts well, it is ready to cut. Cut the curd into 1 cm (½ inch) intervals using a curd cutting knife. Cut from top to bottom and left to right. Next, using a curd cutting rack, cut through horizontally. Allow the curd to rest for 5 minutes.

Turn the curd
Over the next hour, gently turn the curd continuously. While turning the curd, slowly cook the curd, bringing the temperature of the curd up to 39°C (102°F), do this by adding boiling water into the outer container, making it a bain-marie. As the curd starts releasing whey this can be removed, so we are not wasting energy on heating the whey up as well as the curd. In total you will need to remove approximately 3 litres (102 fl oz/12 cups) whey. As the curd firms up you don't need to be so gentle.

Once the curd is firm and approximately the size of a grain of rice, place 3 litres (102 fl oz/12 cups) of cold water into the curd, bringing the temperature of the curd down to 26°C (86°F), and stir for 15 minutes. Remove 3 litres (102 fl oz/12 cups) of the whey, water liquid and replace with the other 3 litres (102 fl oz/12 cups) of cold water from the fridge, dropping the temperature down to 15°C (59°F). Continue turning for a further 15 minutes. Leave the curd to rest for 5 minutes, then drain off as much of the whey as possible.

Hoop the curd
Transfer the curd into an extra large cheese hoop that is lined with cheesecloth, fold the cloth neatly over the curd and place another extra large cheese hoop on top. Press with approximately 4.5 kg (9 lb 14 oz) weight for 30 minutes. Remove from press turn cheese over and rearrange the cheesecloth to minimise creases, then place it back in the hoop with the other hoop on top. Press again overnight with approximately 10 kg (22 lb) weight (some heavy cookbooks will usually do the trick) for 2 hours, then increasing the weight up to 13 kg (28 lb 10 oz) overnight.

Day 2
Remove the cheese from the hoop and cheesecloth and place into a brine bath of 120 g (4¼ oz) non-iodised salt dissolved in 1 litre (35 fl oz/4 cups) of water, using a container that will have the brine solution halfway up the cheese. Leave the cheese in the brine solution for 6 hours turning over after 3 hours, then place on a draining rack to air dry for 24 to 48 hours.

Day 4
When your cheese is feeling dry it is ready to wax. Heat your cheese wax in an old but clean saucepan until just melted. Dip the cheese into the melted wax, making sure it is well covered, usually about three layers of wax is needed to totally seal the cheese.

Store your cheese between 10–15°C (50–59°F) for 4–6 weeks, turning it once a week. Your cheese is then ready to eat!

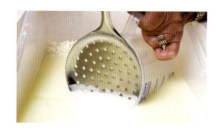
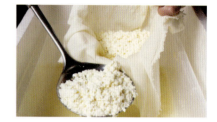
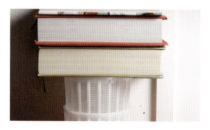
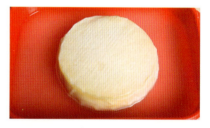
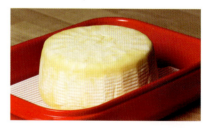
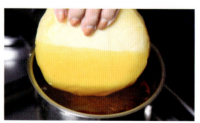

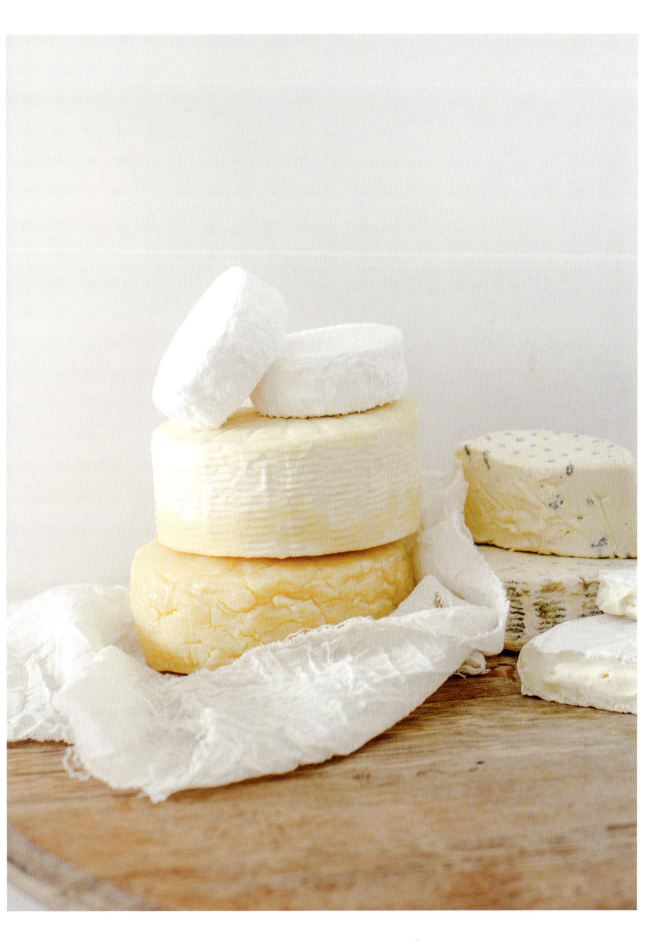

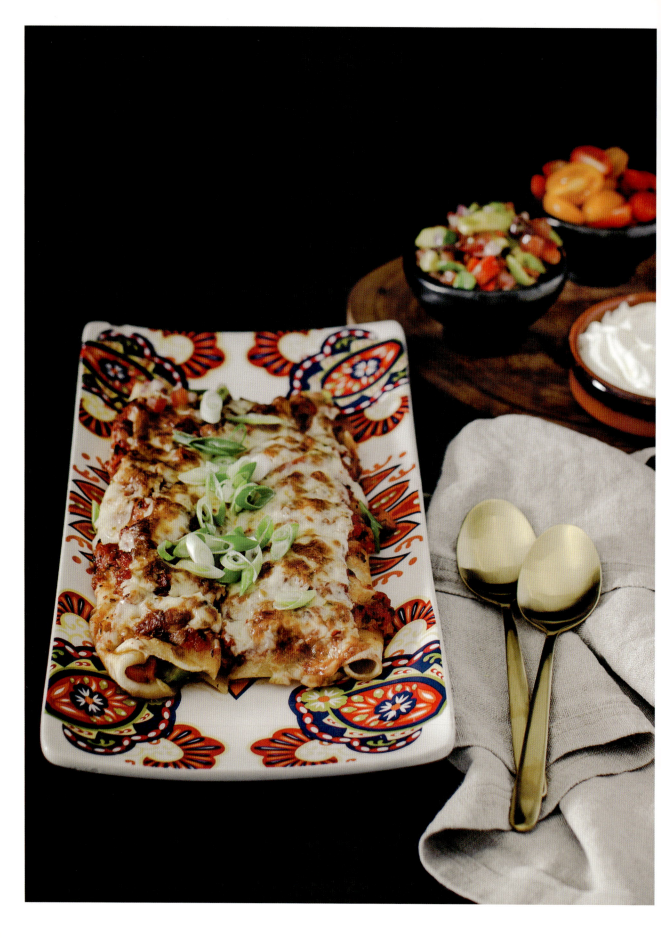

Enchiladas

Serves 6

Flour tortillas
200 g (7 oz) baker's flour
1 teaspoon salt
2 tablespoons oil
125 ml (4 fl oz/½ cup) warm water
oil, for shallow frying

Filling
3 tomatoes, diced
1 red capsicum (bell pepper), chopped
3 avocados, chopped
2 red onions, finely diced
35 g (1¼ oz/¼ cup) chopped olives

Sauce
400 g (14 oz) tinned chopped tomato
1 onion, finely diced
2 garlic cloves, crushed
1 small chilli, seeded and diced
2 teaspoons Mexican spice mix

250 g (7 oz) Monterey Jack cheese, grated
4 spring onions (shallots), sliced

To make the flour tortillas, mix the flour, salt and oil until combined. Add the water and knead for 5 minutes to make a stiff dough. Oil the surface of the dough with a little oil and refrigerate for 1 hour. Divide the dough into six balls, and allow to warm to room temperature. Roll out each ball on a floured surface to a thin 18 cm (7 inch) round. Cover and set aside, until all the tortillas are rolled out.

Meanwhile, make the sauce. Combine all of the ingredients in a bowl and set aside until needed.

Heat the oil in frying pan over medium heat. Add 1 tortilla at a time, for a few seconds, until they begin to blister and become limp, then remove from the oil.

Preheat the oven to 180°C (350°F). Once all tortillas are cooked, fill with the filling and roll to enclose. Place the enchiladas on a baking tray. Top with the sauce and grated Monterey jack. Place in the oven or under the grill (broiler) until the cheese is melted and a little golden. Garnish with sliced spring onions.

Jack & Beans

Serves 4

Polenta
250 g (9 oz) polenta
125 g (4½ oz) grated romano cheese
1 litre (35 fl oz/4 cups) vegetable stock
50 g (1¾ oz) butter
oil, for frying

Beans
400 g (14 oz) tinned red kidney beans
400 g (14 oz) tinned diced tomatoes
1 onion, diced
3 tablespoons tomato paste
½ red capsicum (bell pepper), diced
2 garlic cloves, crushed
4 bay leaves
2 bird's-eye chillies, deseeded, chopped
2 teaspoons cumin
2 teaspoons dried basil
250 ml (9 fl oz/1 cup) stock
1 tablespoon oil

200 g (7 oz) grated Monterey Jack cheese
spring onions (shallots), sliced diagonally, to garnish

To make the polenta, in a heavy-based saucepan add enough cold water to dampen the polenta and leave for 5 minutes. Bring the vegetable stock to the boil and slowly add to the cold polenta. Bring back to the boil, stirring constantly as it will spit! Reduce the heat and cook for 5 minutes. Add the butter and romano. Place in a 20 x 20 cm (8 x 8 inch) square baking dish and spread out evenly. Refrigerate for 1 hour, or until needed. To cook, slice the polenta, then fry in well-oiled pan on all sides until golden.

To make the beans, heat the oil in the pan, then add the onion and sauté. Add the garlic and chilli and cook for 2 minutes. Add the cumin, bay leaves, basil and tomato paste. Cook for a further 5 minutes, stirring to ensure the tomato paste cooks but does not burn. Add the drained kidney beans, tomatoes and stock. Simmer for 10 minutes.

Serve hot with crispy polenta, topped with Monterey Jack and garnished with spring onions.

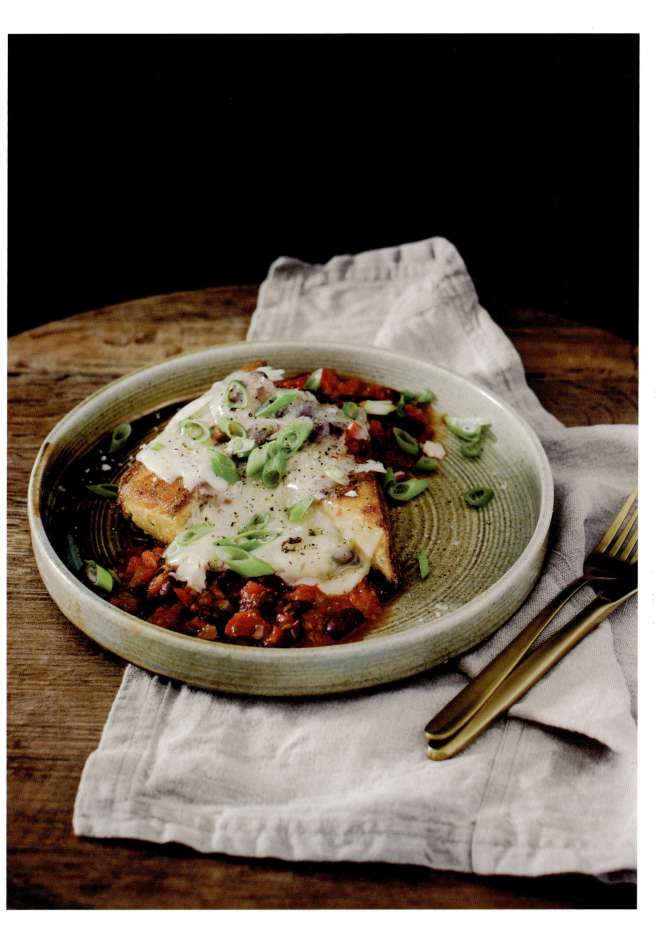

Mozzarella

When I first started making Mozzarella, I was a little confused, whole process was broken down into PH levels and at this point the PH should be this, and at that point the PH level should have dropped to that. My first few attempts were dismal. But, like all cheese, when you think about its origins and the primitive environment it was produced in, you have to think it really can't be that hard. It makes you wonder how did the practice of making a cooked cheese using the Pasta filata or stretched-curd method come about. Maybe someone was making cheese and dropped it into a pot of boiling pasta water. Not wanting to waste it they retrieved it to find it had stretched and was really good on pizza.

This recipe is very simple and if you follow the timing and the temperature, all those worrying PH levels will be fine. I'm quite sure the ancient Romans didn't have a PH testing kit! Mozzarella was originally made using buffalo milk but due to the lac of buffalo in my back paddock, I use cow's milk. The cheese is a creamy, white cheese that should taste of milk. Try not to overwork the curd when turning, as it will make the cheese tough.

Mozzarella

Makes 500 g (1 lb 2 oz) ball

4 litres (135 fl oz/16 cups) un-homogenised milk
1 pinch spoon of type M starter
1 pinch spoon of type T starter
1 pinch spoon of lipase
1 teaspoon citric acid
1 ml (0.03) liquid vegetarian rennet
1 ml (0.03) calcium solution
60 ml (2 fl oz) pre-boiled water, cooled

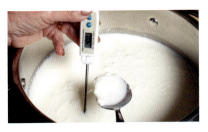

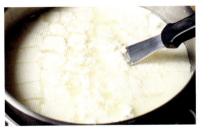

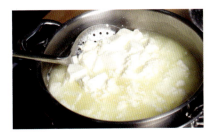

Day 1

Place 1 litre (35 fl oz/4 cups) of water into the fridge to chill. Heat the milk to 35°C (95°F) in a saucepan that will fit into a larger saucepan (we use a double boiler to make the mozzarella). To the warmed milk add the following: type M starter, type T starter, Lipase that has been diluted in 20 ml (½ fl oz) cooled, pre-boiled water and 1 teaspoon of citric acid. Mix in well. Allow the milk to sit for 30 minutes to culture. Mix the calcium solution with 20 ml (½ fl oz) cooled, pre-boiled water and add to the milk. Next, mix the vegetarian rennet with 20 ml (½ fl oz) cool, pre-boiled water. Pour the diluted rennet immediately into the milk, taking care to pour it over as much of the surface as possible. Mix in well and allow the milk to set into a curd. This will take 1 hour.

Cut the curd

Cut the curd into 1.5 cm (⅝ inch) cubes and allow the curd to rest for 20 minutes. Place the smaller saucepan with the curd into a larger saucepan with warm water that comes just to the bottom of the smaller saucepan, creating a double boiler.

Turn the curd

Gently turn the curd while slowly bring the temperature of the curd up to 38°C (100°F), allowing the residual heat from the water in the larger saucepan to bring the final temperature of the curd to 40°C (104°F). This will take approximately 10 minutes.

Rest the curd for 15 minutes, then gently turn. Rest again for 45 minutes. Heat the curd to 43°C (109°F) using the double boiler and remove the whey, maintain the temperature at 43°C (109°F) for the next 2 hours, this will cause the curd to knit together into a single mass.

Turn the mass of curd over every 30 minutes and drain off any excess whey. Remove the small saucepan with the curd from the double boiler and heat the water in the larger saucepan up to 80°C (176°F). You will need to put on a pair of cotton gloves and a pair of new, clean lined washing up gloves as the next part of the mozzarella making is very hot. This step should take approximately 5 minutes. It is called pasta filata, or stretched curd.

Place a small amount of the curd as a test piece into the water at 80°C (176°F) and leave it until it feels slightly melted. Remove it from the water when it has warmed through and gently fold the curd. You can now start to stretch the curd and massage out any lumps. Continue folding and stretching approximately seven times to give a good lamination. A good mozzarella should peel apart once made. Place your stretched curd back into the hot water, allowing it to warm through again. Your curd now needs to be moulded into a ball and placed in cold water from the fridge.

Once you have successfully stretched the test piece, bring the water back up to 80°C (176°F) and repeat the process with the rest of the curd.

Leave the mozzarella in the cold water from the fridge for 1 hour. Then remove it from the cold water and place in a brine solution of 120 g (4¼ oz) of non-iodised salt and 1 litre (35 fl oz/4 cups) of water for 4 hours.

Note
Mozzarella is best eaten fresh but can be cryovaced for up to 1 month stored in the fridge.

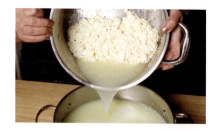
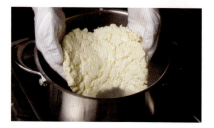
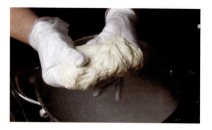
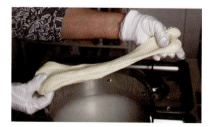
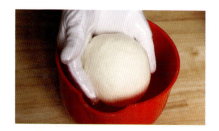
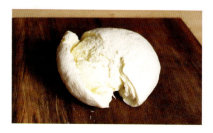

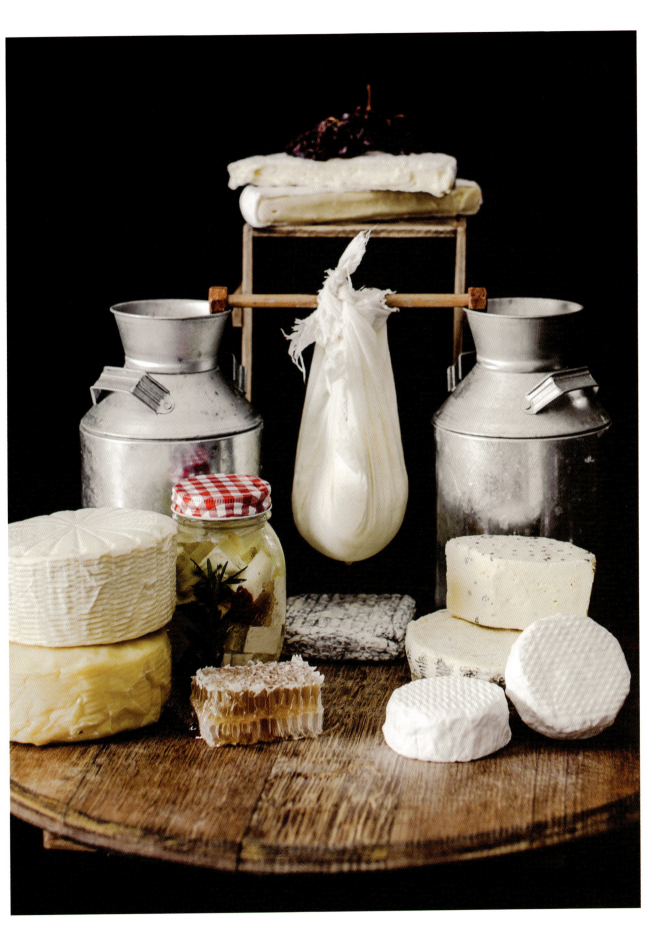

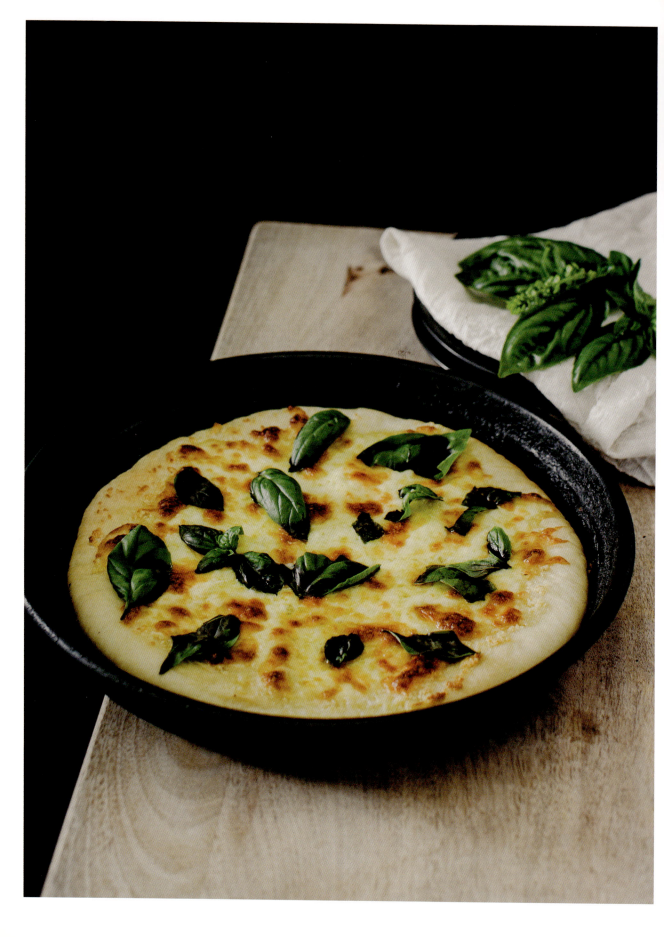

Mozzarella & Basil Pizza

Makes 3 pizzas

Pizza dough
500 g (1 lb 2 oz) baker's flour
2 teaspoon salt
3 teaspoon dried yeast
30 ml (1 fl oz) oil
280 ml (9½ fl oz) warm water

Topping
3 tablespoons olive oil
3 tablespoons finely minced garlic
300 g (10½ oz) mozzarella cheese
50 g (1¾ oz) basil leaves, torn, to garnish

To make the pizza dough, combine all of the ingredients and knead for approximately 10 minutes. Set aside to allow to develop. This will take approximately 1 hour. Knock back and divide the dough into three roll into neat balls. Rest the dough for 5 minutes. Preheat the oven to 200°C (400°F). Roll the dough into thin 25 cm (10 inch) bases. Place the bases on lightly oiled pizza trays.

Spread 1 tablespoon of olive oil onto each base. Add the garlic and top with the mozzarella. Place in the oven for 10 minutes, or until lightly golden. Top with torn basil leaves and serve immediately.

This simple cheese is a real star in a curry. The protein rich paneer served with fresh spinach, combined with a fresh onion and spice paste will have everyone coming back for more. See the Palack Paneer recipe on page 114. Paneer is also a real treat in a pakora batter and fried

The beauty of this cheese is that it can be consume a few hours after it's made, though I find if you refrigerate until cold after pressing it will firm up and be less likely to break up when cooking.

Like ricotta, it can be used either sweet or savory. In India, it is rolled into balls and soaked in a sweet syrup.

Paneer

Makes 300 g (10½ oz)

2 litres (70 fl oz/8 cups) fresh or UHT cow's milk
100 ml (3½ fl oz) lemon juice

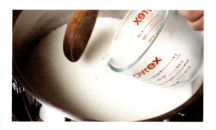

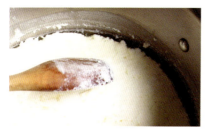

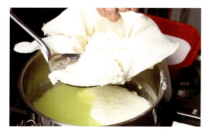

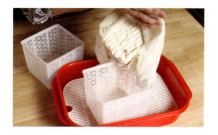

Pour the milk into a large saucepan. Heat the milk, stirring continuously until the milk is almost at the boil, about 94°C (201°F). Add the lemon juice quickly and stir twice around the pot. Remove from the heat. You will notice an instant reaction. The lemon juice will curdle the milk; this creates your curds and whey.

Leave the curds to rest for 20 minutes. During this time the curds will knit into a raft on top of the whey. Using a slotted spoon, scoop the curds gently out of the pot and into a square hoop that has been lined with cheesecloth. Fold the cheesecloth neatly over the curds. Stack another square hoop on top and press with a 4 kg (8 lb 13 oz) weight for 2 hours. (A couple of heavy cookbooks will usually do the trick.)

Place the paneer in the fridge to cool. The Paneer is then ready to consume. It can be stored in an airtight container in the fridge for up to 1 week. Placing it in the fridge will make it firmer for pan-frying.

Palak Paneer Curry

Serves 4

A traditional vegetarian dish originating from the Punjab region of India, the combination of rich, aromatic spices, spinach and cheese make Palak Paneer one of our favorite dishes ...

Curry Paste

3 garlic cloves
1 brown onion, quartered
4 cm (1½ inch) knob of ginger
1 small red chilli
1 teaspoon cumin seeds
1 tablespoon rice bran oil
2 tablespoons tomato paste
1 teaspoon ground turmeric
1 teaspoon garam masala

Curry

1 tablespoon rice bran oil
300 g (10½ oz) homemade paneer, diced
125 ml (4 fl oz/½ cup) stock
440 ml (15¼ fl oz) tinned coconut cream
1 bunch spinach, stalks removed, chopped

steamed rice, to serve
naan bread, to serve
plain yoghurt, to serve
coriander (cilantro), to garnish
squeeze of fresh lemon or lime

To make the curry paste, place the garlic, onion, ginger and chilli in a food processor and blend to a paste. Set aside until needed. Place the cumin seed into a large frying pan with a little oil and cook for about 1 minute over low heat until aromatic. Add the onion, garlic and chilli mix. Increase the heat to medium–high and stir for approximately 2 minutes. Add the tomato paste and continue cooking until the mixture turns a deep red/brown color. Stir in the turmeric and garam masala, then set aside.

To make the curry, heat the oil in a large frying pan over medium heat. Add the paneer and cook until it browns on all sides, then remove from the pan. Place the curry paste back into the pan, with the stock, coconut cream and spinach. Cook until the spinach has wilted, then add the paneer back into the pan. When heated through, remove from the heat.

Serve with steamed rice and naan bread. Add a dollop of yoghurt, garnish with coriander and squeeze over some lemon or lime juice.

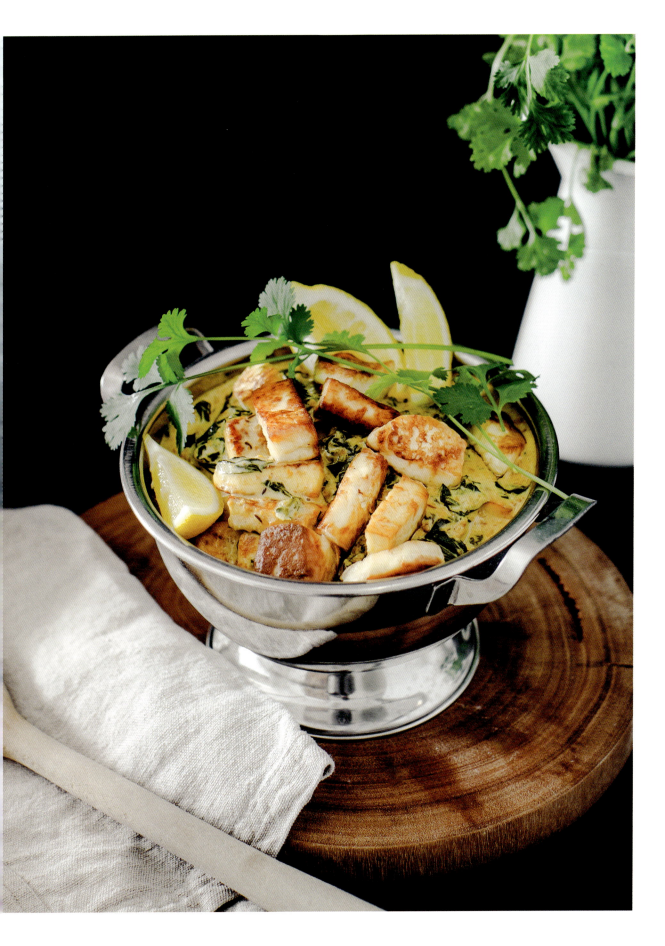

Quark

Quark is a German cheese. It's a fresh cream cheese that can be used anywhere you would use cream cheese. It's used for baking and as a breakfast spread and also forms the basis of a large number of desserts, such as cheesecakes. The large popularity of quark desserts has until recently been limited to European countries. Quark is made by adding a starter culture to milk and incubating it at approximately 40°C (104°F) for a minimum of 10 hours, then strained. It's a soft, white fresh cheese that contains no salt, vegetable gums, preservatives or extra milk solids. It's purely milk and starter.

At only the cost of the milk and pinch or 1/10th teaspoon of culture, your cheesecakes just became so much less expensive to make!

Quark

Makes 250 g (9 oz)

1 litre (35 fl oz/4 cups) UHT milk
1 pinch of Mesophilic starter culture (type M starter)

In a yoghurt pot, combine the type M starter with the UHT milk. Place the pot into a yoghurt maker and incubate for a minimum of 10 hours, and up to 16 hours. Leave it until is has set. Place the inner yoghurt pot into the fridge and allow to chill through completely.

Once chilled, remove the lid from the container and cover with cheesecloth. Holding down the sides tightly, turn the quark out into a colander that is lined with cheesecloth and placed in a jug or bowl, to catch the whey. Tie the opposite corners of the cheesecloth over a wooden spoon and hang over a container in the fridge for 24–48 hours. Remove from the cheesecloth and your quark is ready.

Store in an airtight container in the fridge for up to 1 week.

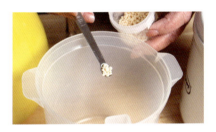
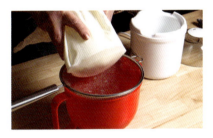
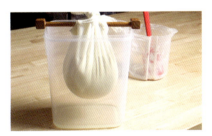
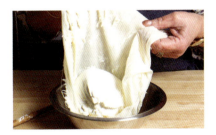

Boursin

Boursin has been made in Normandy, France since its creation in 1963 using fresh milk, cream, cultures, herbs, salt and pepper and other distinctive flavor ingredients. We've been playing with the recipe for our own homemade version of a herb and garlic homemade boursin.

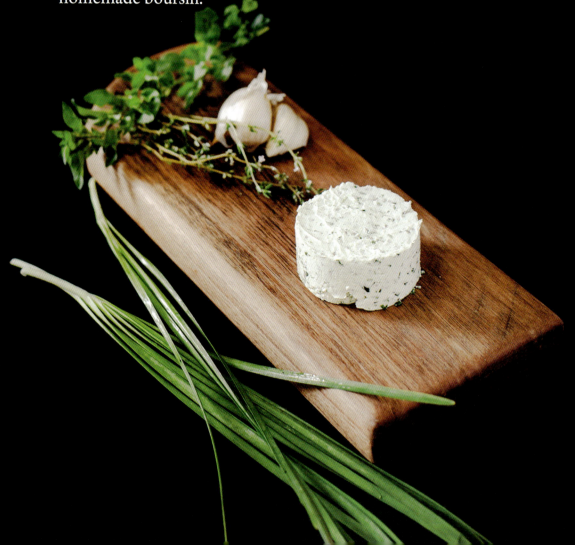

Homemade Boursin

Makes approximately 160 g (5¾ oz)

125 g (4½ oz) quark
30 g (1 oz) fresh finely chopped herbs (such as chives, oregano, thyme)
1 garlic clove, finely grated
pinch of salt

Make sure your homemade quark is well drained, at least 48 hours. If still soft, spread it out on a few layers of good-quality paper towel to draw out excess moisture. The paper towel will just peel off the quark.

Place the quark into a mixing bowl with the herbs, garlic, salt and pepper mix thoroughly. Check the seasoning and adjust to taste.

To shape the quark into a squat cylinder, oil a cookie cutter and pack the quark-boursin into the cookie cutter on your cheese board, then slid the cutter up to remove it from the cheese.

Note
Homemade Boursin can be made up to 2 days in advance, and stored covered in the fridge until ready to use.

Ricotta

The word 'ricotta' simply means 're-cooked'! In mass production cheeseries, the curd needed for cheese making is removed from its whey, then some fresh milk is added to coagulate the remaining protein in the whey. The whey is heated to the boil and an acidifying agent is added to separate the remaining curd from the whey. The curd is collected, drained and ready to use. It's as simple as that!

In our time-poor lifestyles, it isn't practical to make a batch of mozzarella first to then make our ricotta from the whey. So when making ricotta at home, we use full cream milk. I even add an extra 100 ml (3½ fl oz) cream to make it even nicer if I'm after a creamier ricotta. This cheese can be made and eaten within an hour. You'll never buy ricotta again!

Ricotta

Makes 250 g (9 oz)

1 litre (35 fl oz/4 cups) milk (cow or goat)
50 ml (1¾ fl oz) white vinegar

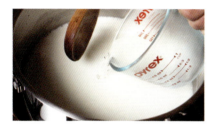

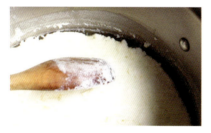

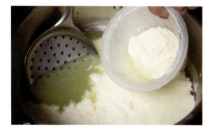

Heat the milk in a heavy based saucepan to a little over 90–94°C (194–201°F), just on the boil, while continuously stirring to avoid the milk burning. When the milk is just on the boil, quickly add the white vinegar. Give it two good stirs, then remove from the heat. Leave to rest for 20 minutes to allow the curd to knit together to form a raft on top of the whey.

Transfer the curd using a slotted spoon into a ricotta hoop and drain for 20 minutes. The ricotta is ready to use immediately or store in an airtight container until required. Fresh ricotta will keep in the fridge for approximately 1 week.

Note

If you prefer a rich creamy ricotta, add 100 ml (3½ fl oz) in addition to the 1 litre (35 fl oz/4 cups) milk. There is no need to adjust the vinegar, this gives a creamier mouth feel and softer ricotta.

Ricotta Gnocchi with Parmesan Broth

Serves 4

The word gnocchi in Italian means 'little lump'. It was originally served as an extra during a traditional Italian meal. Gastronomically speaking however, gnocchi should be anything but lumpish, a well-made gnocchi should be light and fluffy. This parmesan broth is delicious and a great way to use up the parmesan rinds.

Broth

250 g (9 oz/1 cup) parmesan rind, in chunks
1.5 litres (52 fl oz/6 cups) vegetable stock
1 onion, diced
2 garlic cloves, bruised
2 celery stalks, diced
1 carrot, diced
4 bay leaves
2 teaspoons black peppercorns
pinch of salt

Ricotta gnocchi

100 g (3½ oz) plain (all-purpose) flour
250 g (9 oz) ricotta cheese
pinch of grated nutmeg
zest of 1 lemon or lime
pinch of salt

25 g (1 oz) butter
12 sage leaves, to garnish
1 nip of brandy (optional)
shaved parmesan cheese, to serve

To make the broth, place all the ingredients into a saucepan and simmer for approximately 45 minutes, stirring occasionally to make sure the parmesan rind doesn't stick to the bottom of the pot. When the broth is done, strain through a fine sieve or colander and discard the solids. You should end up with approximately 1 litre (35 fl oz/4 cups) broth.

To make the gnocchi, gradually add most of the flour to the ricotta, nutmeg, zest and salt, reserving a little flour. Knead until it becomes a smooth mixture. Once the mixture becomes soft and smooth stop kneading and allow it to rest. Dust work area with a little flour. Divide mixture into four and roll into a sausage. Cut into 1 cm (¾ inch) pieces and roll each piece with the curved side of fork or a gnocchi board. This creates a surface for the broth to stick to the gnocchi. Bring a large pot of water to the boil and add salt. Drop in the gnocchi, in batches, remembering not to overcrowd the pot. When the gnocchi rise to the surface, remove with a slotted spoon, place in a warm oiled baking tray to keep warm and continue cooking remaining gnocchi.

To make the burnt butter sage leaves, heat the butter in a frying pan over medium heat and cook until frothing and nut brown in color. Add the sage leaves and continue cooking until the leaves become crisp. Remove from the pan and place on a paper towel until ready to serve.

When all the gnocchi is cooked, reheat the broth and add a nip of brandy to the broth (optional). Place the warm gnocchi into serving bowls and pour over the broth, garnish with sage and a little shaving of parmesan.

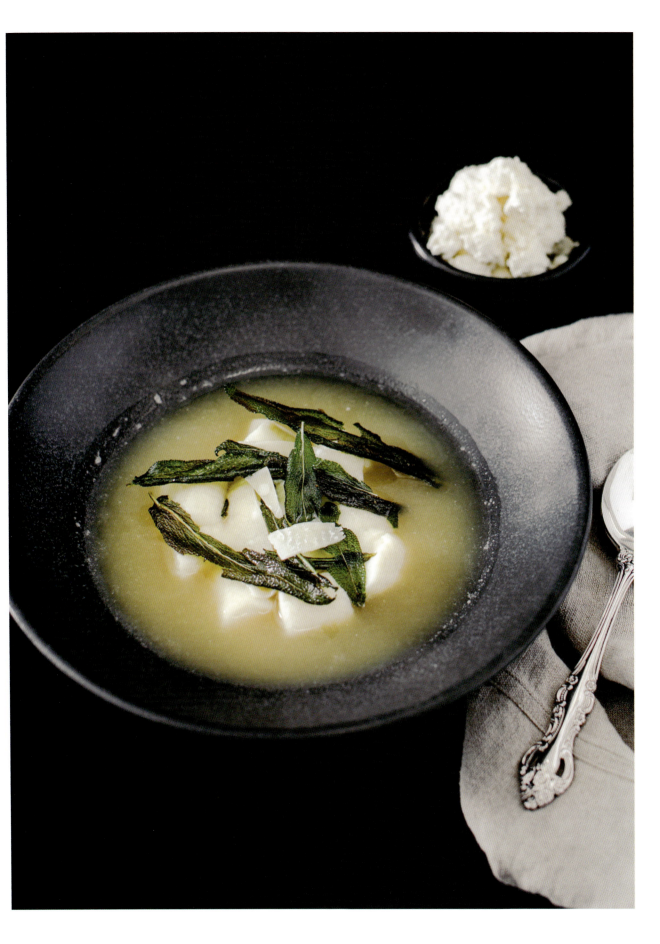

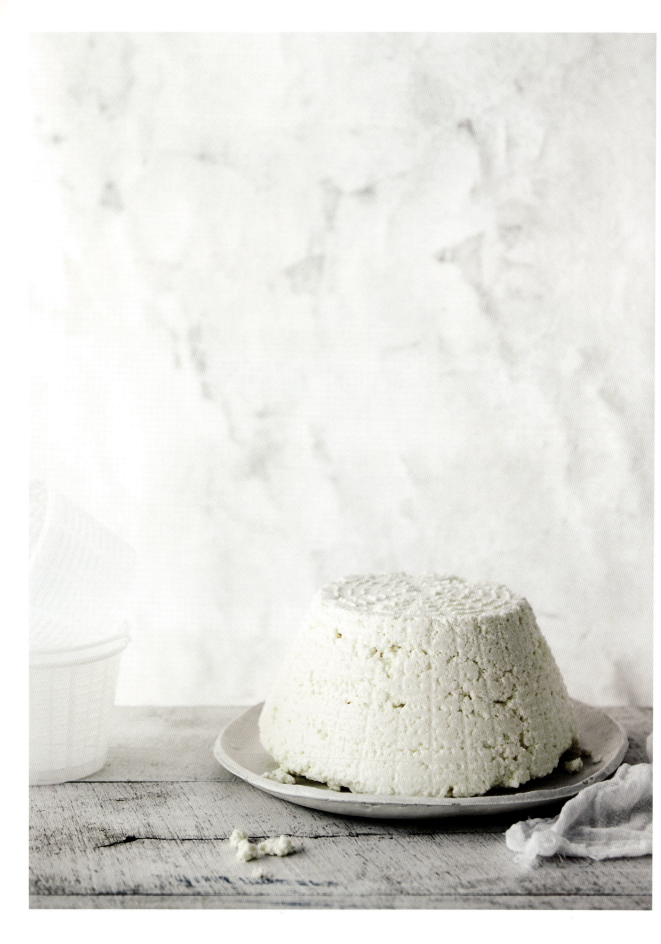

Ricotta Salata (poor man's parmesan)

Makes 275 g (9¾ oz)

2 litres (70 fl oz/8 cups) milk (cow or goat)
100 ml (3½ fl oz) white vinegar
50 g (1¾ oz) salt

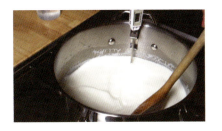

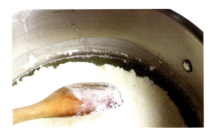

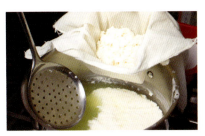

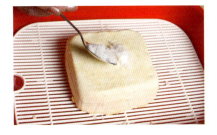

In a heavy-based saucepan, heat the milk to a little over 90–94°C (194–201°F) (just on the boil), while continuously stirring to avoid the milk burning on the bottom of the pot.

When the milk is just on the boil, quickly add the white vinegar. Give it two good stirs, then remove from the heat. Leave for 20 minutes for the curd to form a raft on top of the whey.

Transfer the curd using a slotted spoon, placing the curd into a square hoop lined with cheesecloth. Place another square hoop on top and press with approximately 4 kg (8 lb 13 oz) weight (a couple of heavy book will do) for 20 minutes. Then turn the curd over and rearrange the cheesecloth to smooth out any creases. Press again for approximately 1 hour.

Remove the cheese from the hoop and store, uncovered, in the fridge for 24 hours. For the next 7 days, rub a pinch of salt into the outside of the cheese once daily. The cheese should be stored in the fridge at all times (I leave the lid off to assist with the drying of the cheese). After 7 days your cheese is ready for eating and can be stored for up to 7 weeks.

Baked Ricotta Custard

Serves 12

500 g (1 lb 2 oz) ricotta cheese
125 ml (4 fl oz/½ cup) pure cream
125 ml (4 fl oz/½ cup) milk
4 eggs
4 teaspoons cornflour (cornstarch)
2 teaspoons vanilla bean paste
125 g (4½ oz) caster (superfine) sugar

Preheat the oven to 140°C (275°F).

Put all of the ingredients into a food processor or blender and process until smooth. Transfer the mixture into a jug with a pouring lip for easy pouring.

Place a lightly greased silicone muffin pan onto a baking tray that will hold a little water. Pour the mixture into the silicone muffin pan holes. Pour 250 ml (9 fl oz/1 cup) water into the baking tray that the muffin pan is sitting on.

Bake for 20 minutes, or until they are firm when the tray is wobbled or a skewer comes out clean. When cool, and while still in the muffin pan, place in the fridge or freezer to completely cool before removing from the muffin holes.

Notes

Serve the individual baked ricotta custards with some whipped ricotta chocolate mouse, sweetened mascarpone, strawberries and strawberry coulis.

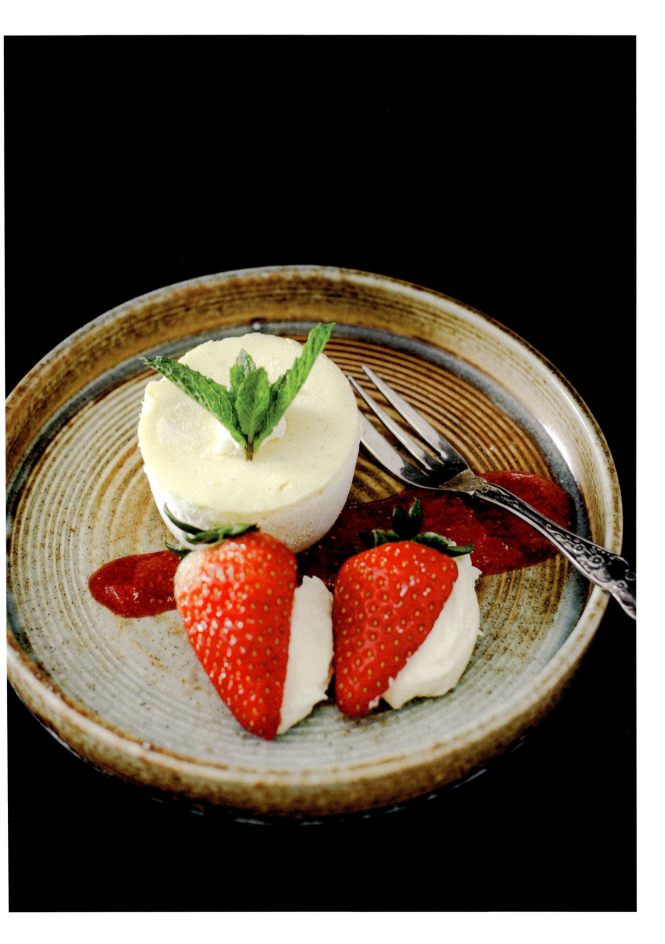

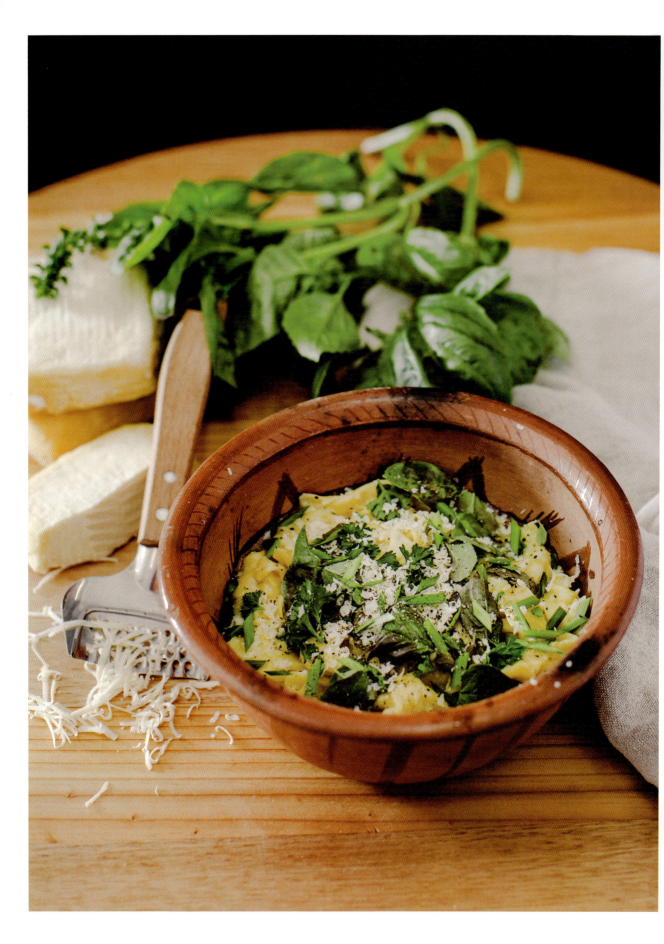

Rag Pasta with Poor Man's Parmesan

Serves 4

Pasta
250 g (9 oz) '00' flour
2 eggs
3 egg yolks

Sauce
75g (3 oz) butter
1 garlic clove, crushed
2 teaspoons stock powder
150 ml (5 fl oz) pasta water

50 g (1¾ oz) ricotta salata
fresh herbs, to garnish
salt and pepper, to season

Pasta – Method by hand
Place the flour on the workbench and make a well in the centre. Lightly whisk the eggs and place in a well. Using a knife, bring the eggs and flour together. If the mixture is too dry, add 1 teaspoon of water. Knead for approximately 10 minutes, or until firm and smooth. Cover and set aside to rest for 10 minutes.

Method with mixmaster
Place the flour and egg into bowl and using the dough hook attachment, bring the flour and egg together. If too dry, add 1 teaspoon of water. Once the flour and egg is combined, knead for 10 minutes. Don't leave the machine as it's quite hard work for it. Rest the pasta for 10 minutes. Cut the dough into four fingers and feed through the pasta machine starting at the widest setting 0. Feed the dough through this setting three times, then fold the pasta into thirds and pass through the 0 "wide" setting 3 times. Fold into thirds again and roll three times again on 0. Then you can reduce the setting to 1 (no more folding), just pass the dough through the roller three times. Reduce the setting to 2. Put the dough through this setting three times and continue until you are down to setting number 5. This is a good thickness for lasagne and fettuccini. If you require a finer pasta, reduce the setting further. Cut your pasta into random shapes.

Bring a large saucepan of water to the boil. Place the pasta into boiling water and simmer for approximately 3 minutes, or until al dente.

Melt the butter in a large enough pan to toss the pasta in. Add the garlic and cook for 1 minute. Mix the stock powder with the pasta water to dissolve, then add the stock to the butter and garlic. Toss the pasta through the butter, season with salt and pepper and garnish with fresh herbs and grated ricotta salata.

Romano

The Romans were passionate about cheese, both eating it and making it. Romano, named after the Romans, has a variety of types depending on its source. For example, cheese made from sheep's milk is referred to as Pecorino Romano. When made from cow's milk, it's called Vacchino Romano and when made from goat's milk, it's called Caprino Romano.

Romano is a sharp, dry cheese that is suitable for grating and can be used as a substitute for parmesan.

Romano

Makes 900 g (2 lb)

8 litres (270 fl oz) non-homogenised milk
1 pinch spoon of type T starter
1 pinch spoon lipase
2.5 ml (0.08 fl oz) liquid vegetarian rennet
125 g (4½ oz) non-iodised salt
1 litre (35 fl oz/4 cups) water
45 ml (1½ fl oz) boiled water, cooled

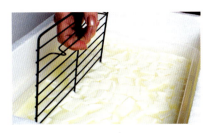

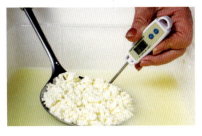

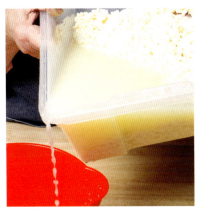

Day 1

In a large saucepan heat the non-homogenised milk to 32°C (89°F). Once warm transfer the milk into your cheese vat. Add the type T starter, to the milk. Add the lipase to 20 ml (½ fl oz) boiled water, cooled. Stir and pour into the warm milk. Mix thoroughly. Leave the milk to culture for 1 hour.

Mix the liquid vegetarian rennet with 25 ml (1 fl oz) cool, pre-boiled water. Pour the rennet immediately into the milk, taking care to pour it over as much of the surface as possible. Mix in well and allow the milk to set into a curd. This will take 40 minutes.

Cut the curd

To check the curd, place the blade of a curd cutting knife into the curd and lift at a 45-degree angle, looking for a clean break. If the curd parts well, it is ready to cut. Cut the curd into 1cm (½ inch) intervals using a curd cutting knife. Cut from top to bottom and left to right. Next, using a curd cutting rack, cut through horizontally. Allow the curd to rest for 5 minutes.

Turn the curd

Over the next hour, gently turn the curd continuously. While turning the curd, slowly cook the curd, bringing the temperature of the curd up to 48°C (118°F), do this by adding boiling water into the styrene box that the cheese vat is sitting in, making it a bain-marie.

As the curd starts releasing whey this can be removed, so we are not wasting energy on heating the whey up as well as the curd. In total you will need to remove approximately 3 litres (102 fl oz/12 cups) of whey. As the curd firms up you don't need to be so gentle, you will have to constantly turn the curd as it will start to knit together as it warms up. Once the curd is firm and approximately the size of a grain of rice, leave the curd to rest for 5 minutes, then drain off as much of the whey as possible.

Transfer the curd into an extra large cheese hoop that is lined with cheesecloth. Fold the cloth neatly over the curd and place another extra large cheese hoop on top. Press with approximately 8 kg (17 lb 10 oz) weight for 30 minutes. Remove the curd from press turn cheese over and rearrange the cheesecloth to minimise creases, then place it back in the hoop with the other hoop on top. Press again with approximately 10 kg (22 lb) weight for 1 hour (Some heavy cookbooks will usually do the trick). While pressing the curd you need to maintain a temperature of approximately 30°C (86°F) do this by wrapping it in a clean towel. Remove the curd from the press, turn the cheese over and rearrange the cheesecloth to minimise creases, then place it back in the hoop with the other hoop on top. Press again with approximately 20 kg (44 lb) weight overnight.

Day 2

Remove the cheese from the hoop and cheesecloth. Make up a brine solution of 300 g (10½ oz) non-iodised salt and 1 litre (35 fl oz/4 cups) water, making sure the brine comes half way up the curd. The curd needs to be brined for 4 hours turning it over after 2 hours. Remove from the brine solution and place on a draining rack to air dry, at room temperature.

Day 4

When your cheese is feeling dry it is ready to wax. Heat your cheese wax in an old but clean saucepan until just melted. Dip the cheese into the melted wax, making sure it is well covered, usually about three layers of wax is needed to totally seal the cheese. Store your cheese at 10–15°C (50–59°F) for 3 to 12 months, turning it once a week.

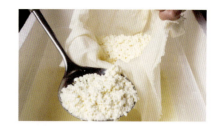
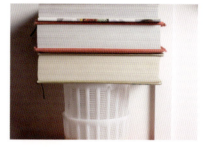
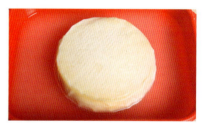
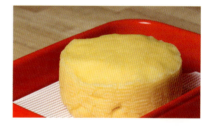
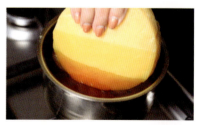
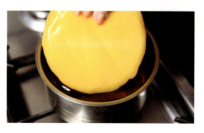

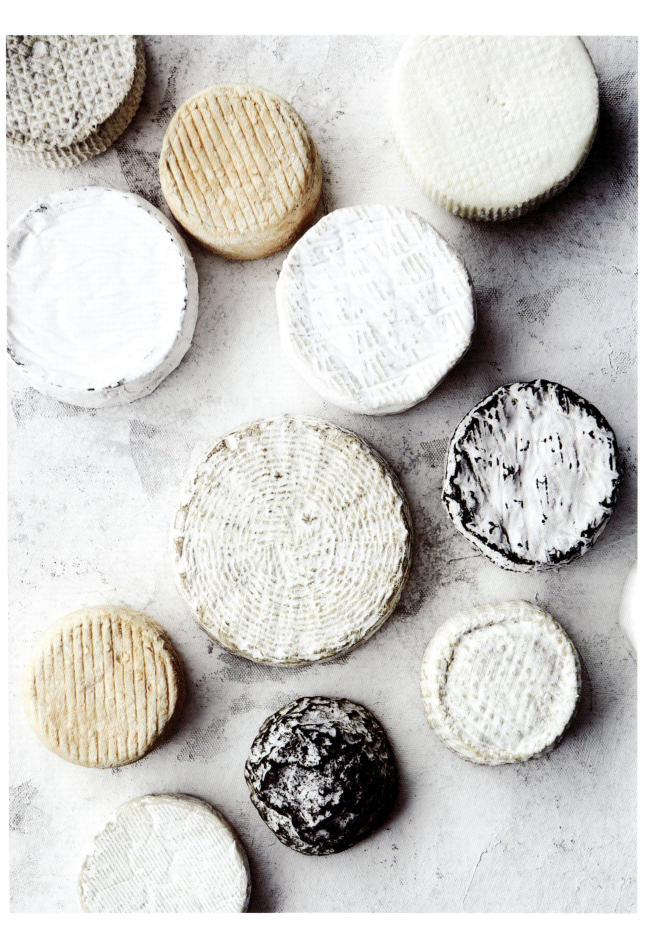

Washed Rind

Washed rind cheeses can have totally different flavors depending on what they have been washed in. Brevy linens or Brevibacterium linens gives washed rind cheeses their sticky orange surface, and an earthy aroma. I have used things like Grand Marnier to give my cheese a real punch of flavor, Champagne, beer or wine can also be used. The washing of the rind of the cheese as it matures keeps it soft and supple, as it develops its own unique flavor. It may not be the prettiest of cheese, it is probably the smelliest but it makes up for this by being delicious. A washed rind cheese is best eaten when fully ripe and always served at room temperature. Try serving on a slice of toasted sourdough and a medium-bodied shiraz or a cold beer.

This style of cheese has been made in Europe since the Middle Ages.

Washed Rind

Makes 2 x 200 g (7 oz)

4 litres (135 fl oz/16 cups) non-homogenised milk
1 pinch spoon of type T type starter
1.2 ml (0.04 fl oz) liquid vegetarian rennet
20 ml (½ fl oz) pre-boiled water, cooled
200 g (7 oz) non-iodised salt
20 g (¾ oz) non-iodised salt
1 drop spoon of brevy linens

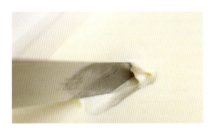

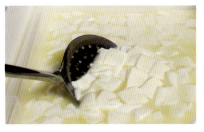

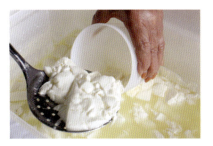

Day 1
In a large saucepan, heat the non-homogenised milk to 42°C (107.6°F). Once warmed, transfer the milk into your cheese vat. To your milk, add the type T starter. Leave for 45 minutes.

Mix the rennet with the cooled pre-boiled water. Pour the rennet immediately into the milk, taking care to pour it over as much of the surface as possible. Mix in well and allow the milk to set into a curd. This will take 40 minutes.

Cut the curd
To check the curd, place the blade of a knife into the curd and lift at a 45-degree angle, looking for a clean break. If the curd parts well, it is ready to cut. Cut the curd in 2.5 cm (1 inch) intervals using a curd cutting knife. Cut from top to bottom and left to right. Next, using a curd cutting rack to cut through horizontally. Allow curd to rest for 5 minutes.

Turn the curd
Using a curd turning spoon, slide the spoon down the side of the vat and underneath the curd. Then gently lift and jiggle, bringing the curd turning spoon to the surface. Continue until all of the curd has been turned once. Rest curd for 30 minutes and gently turn again. Rest curd again for another 30 minutes and turn again. The curd will need to be turned three times total.

Draining the whey
Taking a curd turning spoon and a plastic jug again, drain off as much of the whey as possible. Then using a curd turning spoon, ladle the curd into medium cheese hoops, filling to the top. Once filled, the hoops need to be placed onto a draining tray. Cover the hoops with cheesecloth and rest for 5 minutes. Invert the hoop by holding onto

the cheesecloth and turning over. Continue to invert hoop five times over the next 3 to 4 hours and drain off any excess whey as you go. Leave the curd in the hoop overnight at room temperature.

Day 2

The next morning, make a brine solution using 200 g (7 oz) non-iodised salt and 1 litre (35 fl oz/4 cups) water. Remove the curd from the hoops and place into the cooled brine solution. Leave the cheese for 30 minutes, turn over, then leave for another 30 minutes. Remove the curd from the brine solution and place on a draining rack for 24 to 48 hours at room temperature with no lid on. Turn the cheese every 12 hours to make sure they dry evenly, removing any whey from the draining rack container.

Once your cheeses feel clammy, not wet, place a lid on to drying rack container to create a humid environment. Store the cheese between 10–15°C (50–59°F) for 14 days.

While your cheese is maturing you will need to start to wash it. Make a weak brine solution of 20 g (¾ oz) non-iodised salt with 500 ml (17 fl oz) cold, pre-boiled water. Stir until salt is dissolved and add a drop spoon of brevi linens. Wash the cheese every second day with the same solution, for 2 weeks. The cheese needs to be turned second day as well. The wash will get a quite smelly but the end result is delicious.

Wrap your cheese in baking paper then foil and store in the fridge at 4°C (39.2°F). It is ready to start enjoying immediately and will get stronger the longer it is left.

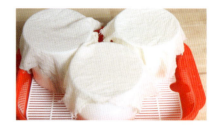
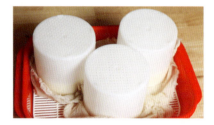
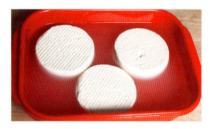
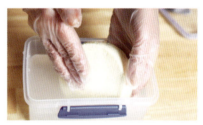
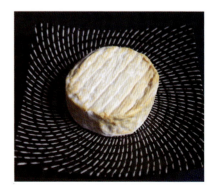

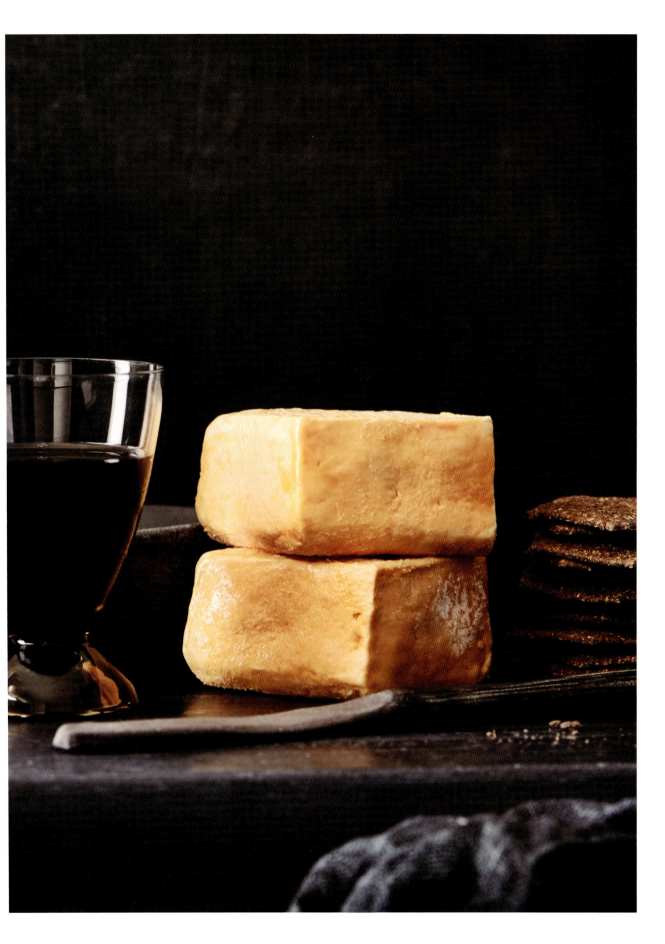

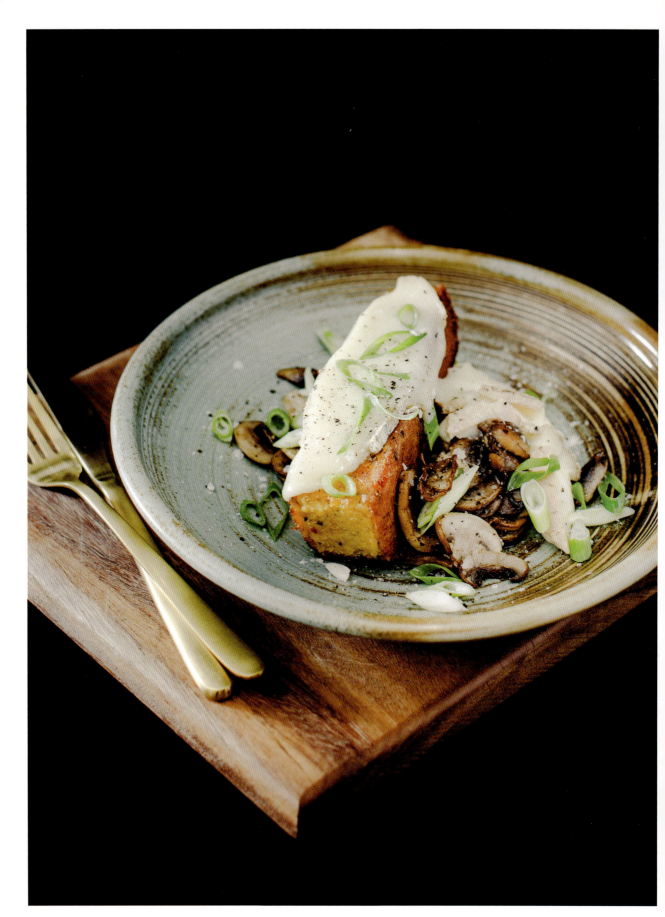

Fried Polenta and Mushrooms with Washed Rind

Serves 4

150 g (5½ oz) fine polenta
500 ml (17 fl oz/2 cups) vegetable stock
1 teaspoon salt
2 teaspoons dried Italian herbs
50 g (1¾ oz) chopped butter
100 g (3½ oz) grated romano cheese
vegetable oil, for shallow frying
500 g (1 lb 2 oz) sliced mushrooms
4 garlic cloves, crushed
100 g (3½ oz) sliced washed rind cheese
finely sliced spring onions (shallots), to garnish

Place the polenta in a heavy-based saucepan. Add enough water to moisten and leave for 5 minutes.

Place the vegetable stock in a separate saucepan and bring to the boil. Gradually pour the stock into the polenta. Add the herbs and cook over low heat, stirring constantly, until it comes away from the sides of the pot. Add the butter and romano and stir thoroughly. Place hot polenta immediately into a greased loaf tin. Smooth the top and refrigerate until set which will take approximately 1 hour. Remove from the loaf pan and slice into 3 cm (1½ inches) thick slices and set aside.

Meanwhile, heat a small amount of oil in a large frying pan. Add the garlic and mushrooms. Stir until they begin to color, then add the remaining butter. Stir until golden. Season to taste. Place in an ovenproof dish and keep warm.

Heat the vegetable oil in pan over high heat and cook the polenta slices until golden and crisp. Divide into four serves by placing mushrooms in the centre of the plate, top with the polenta and sliced washed rind cheese, then garnish with shallots. Serve immediately.

Yoghurt

The word yoghurt comes from Turkey. Yoghurt is fermented milk, probably discovered accidentally by milk being kept in warm climates with no refrigeration. The naturally occurring bacteria in the milk converts the milk to yoghurt which changes both the flavor and texture. It wasn't long before the health benefits of yoghurt were realised. We use a ABY Probiotic yoghurt culture to make our Greek-style yoghurt. It is smooth, creamy and just a little sharp, whereas the ABT Probiotic yoghurt culture is missing that sharp note, which makes it a little more kid friendly.

Greek Yoghurt

Makes 1 kg (2 lb 4 oz)

1 litre (35 fl oz/4 cups) UHT milk
4 dessertspoons milk powder
1 pinch ABY probiotic yoghurt culture or ABT for a milder yoghurt

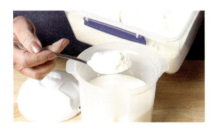

In a yoghurt container, add the milk, milk powder and ABY probiotic yoghurt culture. Mix in thoroughly. Incubate in your yoghurt maker for a minimum of 10 hours.

Remove the container from the yoghurt maker. Place the container in the fridge and allow to chill through completely. Once cooled, your yoghurt is ready for eating.

Note
Your yoghurt will remain fresh for up to 1 week.

Labne

Makes 500 g (1 lb 2 oz)

1 kg (2 lb 4 oz) ready-made Greek yoghurt
salt, to taste
minced garlic, to taste (optional)
fresh herbs or lime zest, to garnish

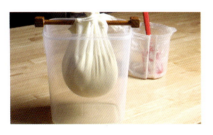

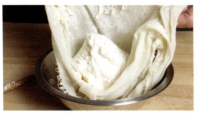

Remove the lid from the container of yoghurt and cover with cheesecloth. Holding the cheesecloth tightly, turn the container upside down into a colander that is sitting in a jug or bowl. Tie the opposing corners of the cheesecloth over a wooden spoon and hang over a container for 48 hours.

Fold through the salt, garlic plus your choice of seasoning and place labne into an airtight container.

Note
If you are using your labne as a fresh spread, it will remain fresh in the fridge for up to 1 week if kept in an airtight container. Alternatively, you can spread your labne out on good quality paper towel to absorb more moisture then, roll your seasoned labne into balls and cover in sunflower oil. It will keep for up to 1 month in the fridge covered with the oil.

Tzatziki

Serves 6

250 g (8¾ oz) labne
1 Lebanese (short) cucumber, peeled, deseeded and grated
2 garlic cloves
1 small handful mint leaves
salt and pepper, to season

Salt the grated cucumber and leave to stand for 5 minutes to draw out liquid. Squeeze out the cucumber and place into the labne.

Grate the garlic using a fine microplane. Add to the labne. Finely chop the mint leaves and add to labne. Mix thoroughly and refrigerate until needed. Serve as a dip.

Note
May be stored in an airtight container in the fridge for up to 4 days, but is best eaten fresh.

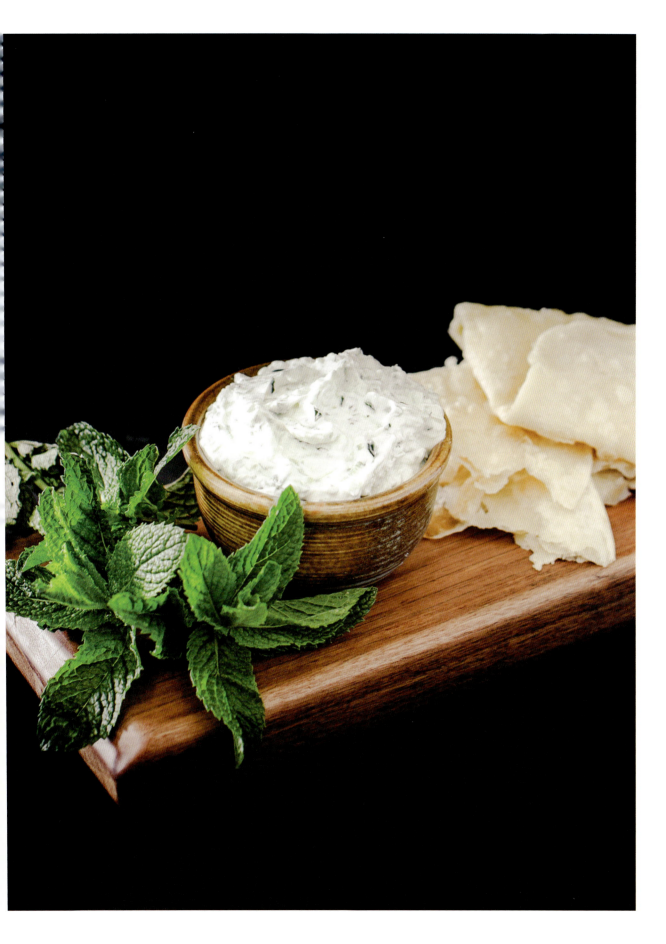

Goat Cheese

Before reading this book, you may have thought that making cheese would be complicated, and there seems to be even more mystery about the art of making goat's cheese. The reasons for this, I don't understand. Perhaps it's that in Australia, goat milk hasn't been as readily available as cow. Yet goat's cheese has been around for centuries.

In the pages that follow, I have included a few of the recipes from the previous pages and just 'tweaked' them a little to give you delicious goat's cheese. Once you have started making your own goat's cheese, you can become more adventurous and try many of the recipes in this book using goat's milk, just by adding calcium solution at the same rate and time as rennet. You'll need a little bit more patience and remember to be super gentle with the curd, as it is quite delicate.

It is always best to use the milk as fresh as possible as it is less 'goaty' in taste. Also milking goats that are in a paddock with a buck will have a stronger, 'goaty' taste to the milk. One of my very dear friends, Jenny, has the most beautiful Saanen dairy goats which she uses to make 'Divine Goats Milk Soap'. Using her milk to make cheese, I get the most delicate flavor. We also have a Boer Goat producer locally and when making cheese using his milk, I get a far more robust cheese. The breed of the animal and the pasture they are grazing on makes a huge difference.

Goat's cheese, with its pristine white color and distinct flavor, is one of the most amazing foods. Humble and basic for some and gourmet for others. It can range in taste from strong and pungent, to delicate and mild. It also varies in texture from creamy, to semi firm, to crumbly.

Chèvre

Makes 2 x 500 g (1 lb 2 oz)

Chèvre is the french word for goat and is often used to describe a soft goat cheese, the following recipe is for a fresh chèvre which is a soft cream cheese that is delicious in salads or served with bread, olives, tomato and basil. Goat's milk is non-homogenised as the fat molecules in the goat milk are so small that there is no need to homogenise it. Lactose intolerant people often find goat's cheese a better option in their diet as it is easier to digest.

Did you know ...

You can easily make your own ash! Grab some baby grapevine leaves or fresh basil from your garden. Put them in a heavy-based saucepan and burn them, they become ash!

You can ash goat's chèvre by using this simple technique: Lay out a sheet of plastic wrap. Place enough ash to coat half of the cheese log, then top with chèvre. Sprinkle with more ash to cover the cheese. Using the plastic wrap, roll the ash and chèvre until it is a cylindrical shape. Twist each end of the plastic wrap to tighten the log.

Another idea: mix chives through the cheese, then roll in parsley or cracked pepper.

4 litres (135 fl oz/16 cups) goat's milk
1 pinch of type M culture
1 ml (0.03 fl oz) liquid vegetarian rennet
1 ml (0.03 fl oz) liquid calcium solution
40 ml (1½ fl oz) boiled water, cooled
60 g (2¼ oz) non-iodised salt

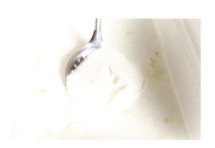

Pour the milk into a large saucepan and heat milk to 25°C (77°F). Once warmed, transfer the milk into your cheese vat. Add the type M culture and liquid calcium solution to 20 ml (½ fl oz) cooled boiled water. Pour the diluted calcium solution over the surface of the milk and stir thoroughly.

Add the liquid vegetarian rennet to 20 ml (½ fl oz) cooled boiled water. Pour the diluted rennet over the surface of the milk and stir thoroughly. Leave for milk to set into a curd. This will take 4 hours. To check the curd, place the blade of a knife into the curd and lift at a 45-degree angle, looking for a clean break. If the curd parts well it is ready.

Transfer the curd into a cheesecloth lined colander sitting over a jug or bowl, to catch the whey and leave it to sit for 6 hours. Tie opposite corners of the cheesecloth over a wooden spoon and hang in a container in the fridge for 24 hours. Remove from the cheesecloth and your fresh chèvre is ready for eating! Store your fresh chevre in an airtight container in the fridge. Your fresh chèvre will last in the fridge for up to 2 weeks.

Goat's Milk Fetta

Makes 2 x 325 g (11 ½ oz) pieces

4 litres (135 fl oz/16 cups) goat milk
1 pinch of type M starter
1 ml (0.03 fl oz) liquid calcium solution
1 ml (0.03 fl oz) liquid vegetarian rennet
40 ml (1½ fl oz) boiled water, cooled
120 g (4¼ oz) non-iodised salt

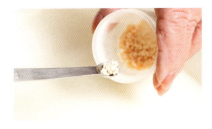

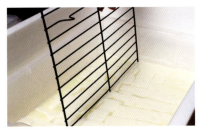

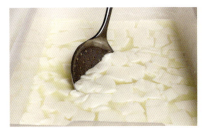

Day 1
In a large saucepan, heat the goat milk to 32°C (89°F). Once warmed, transfer the milk into your cheese vat. Add the type M starter to the milk. Mix the liquid calcium solution to 20 ml (½ fl oz) cooled boiled water, stir and pour into the warm milk. Mix the liquid vegetarian rennet with 20 ml (½ fl oz) cooled, pre-boiled water. Pour the rennet immediately into the milk, taking care to pour it over as much of the surface as possible. Mix in well. Leave the milk to rest for 1.5 hours and the milk will set into a curd.

Cut the curd
To check the curd, place the blade of a knife into the curd and lift at a 45-degree angle, looking for a clean break. If the curd parts well, it is ready to cut. Cut the curd in 1.5 cm (⅝ inch) intervals using a curd cutting knife. Cut from top to bottom and left to right. Next, using a curd cutting rack to cut through horizontally. Allow curd to rest for 5 minutes.

Turn the curd
Using a curd turning spoon, slide the spoon down the side of the vat and underneath the curd. Then gently lift and jiggle, bringing the curd turning spoon to the surface. Continue until all of the curd has been turned once. Rest for an hour and turn for the second time. Rest the curd for an hour then turn for the third time. Rest the curd for 10 minutes. The curd needs to be turned a total of three times.

Draining the whey
Using a curd turning spoon and a plastic jug, place the curd turning spoon over the mouth of the jug and press into the curds so the whey can seep through the spoon to gently drain off as much of the whey as possible.

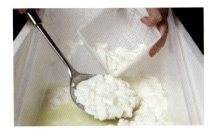
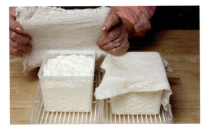
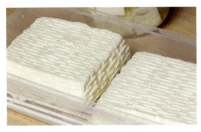
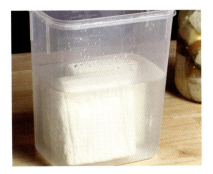

Hooping the curd

Then using a curd turning spoon place the curd into the square cheese hoops, filling each hoop to the top. Do not go back and top up cheese hoops until you have filled both hoops. (They sink down quickly.) Once filled, the hoops need to be placed onto draining trays. Cover the hoops with cheesecloth. Invert the hoops by holding onto the cheesecloth and turning each hoop over. Continue to invert hoops five times over the next 3 to 4 hours and drain off any excess whey as you go. Leave the fetta curd in the hoops overnight at room temperature.

Day 2

Take the fetta out of the cheese hoops and air dry for up to 2 days on a draining rack at room temperature. Turn the cheese morning and night, draining off the whey each time.

Day 3 or 4

Make up a brine solution by adding 120 g (4¼ oz) of non-iodised salt to 1 litre (35 fl oz/4 cups) of boiling water and allow to cool. Put the fetta in the cold brine solution; make sure the brine covers the cheeses. The fetta is ready to consume after 24 hours of being in the brine. It can be stored in brine, in the fridge for 3 months, you will need to replace the brine solution every 3 weeks.

Note

If you want to marinate your fetta, this can be done after the cheese has been in the brine for 24 hours. Place your cheese in a clean, sterile jar with flavors of your choice. We use a bruised garlic clove or chilli, herbs and peppercorns are also good. Make sure the cheese is totally covered in oil. We use sunflower oil as it does not solidify.

Goat's Milk Havarti

Makes 6 x 150 g (5½ oz) pieces

Our Goat's havarti is a semi-hard cheese that can be eaten very young, around 2 weeks after you make it. It can be stored for up to 3 months but it is best eaten young to avoid the taste getting too 'goaty'. It is a moist, smooth cheese that will add a 'wow' factor to your platter. This is a great cheese for anyone lactose intolerant. Not too strong with a nice creamy texture, a really delicious cheese.

8 litres (270 fl oz) goat's milk
1 pinch of type M starter
2.5 ml (0.08 fl oz) liquid calcium solution
2.5 ml (0.08 fl oz) liquid vegetarian rennet
50 ml (1 fl oz) boiled water, cooled
200 g (7 oz) non-iodised salt
2 litres (70 f oz/8 cups) water, chilled

Day 1

In a large saucepan heat the goat's milk to 33°C (91°F). Once warm, transfer the milk into your cheese vat. Add the type M starter to the milk. Mix the liquid calcium solution with 25 ml (1 fl oz) cool, pre-boiled water. Pour the calcium solution immediately into the milk. Mix the liquid vegetarian rennet with 25 ml (1 fl oz) cool, pre-boiled water. Pour the rennet immediately into the milk, taking care to pour it over as much of the surface as possible. Mix in well and allow the milk to set into a curd. This will take 1 hour.

Cut the curd

To check the curd, place the blade of a curd cutting knife into the curd and lift at a 45-degree angle, looking for a clean break. If the curd parts well, it is ready to cut. Cut the curd into 2.5 cm (1 inch) intervals using a curd cutting knife. Cut from top to bottom and left to right. Next, using a curd cutting rack, cut through horizontally. Allow the curd to rest for 5 minutes.

Turn the curd

Over the next 20 minutes gently start to turn the curd. With havarti, you need to be extra gentle, so VERY gently, lifting and jiggling the curd. This will be enough movement to start encouraging whey to be released.

Draining the whey

Using a curd turning spoon and a plastic jug, place the curd turning spoon over the mouth of the jug and press into the curds so the whey can seep through the spoon to gently remove 2 litres (70 fl oz/8 cups) whey.

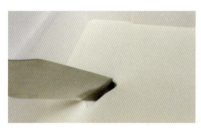
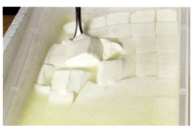

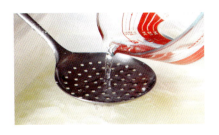

Cooking the curd

Replace the 2 litres (70 fl oz/8 cups) whey with 2 litres (70 fl oz/8 cups) water at 65°C (149°F). Pour the water through your slotted spoon to distribute it evenly without upsetting the curd. Gently move the curd around bringing the temperature of the curd up to 38° (100.4°F). Over the next hour gently, turn the curd around every 10 minutes.

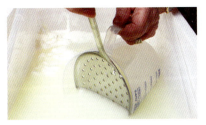

Cooling the curd

Remove 4 litres (135 fl oz/16 cups) whey and replace with the 2 litres (70 fl oz/8 cups) cold water from the fridge, bringing the temperature of the curd down to 28°C (82.4°F). Let the curd rest for 5 minutes then drain off all the whey and briefly and gently turn the curd to encourage a little more whey from the curd. Place the curd into hoops and place another hoop on top. Weigh the hoop down to press with approximately 4 kg (8 lb 13 oz) for 5 minutes, then invert the curd in the hoops and press again for 5 minutes, this is all the pressing required for this cheese. Over the next 2 hours invert the hoops four times. Place the water into a vessel that will hold all the curd and ensure it will come halfway up the side of the curd. Place the vessel of water into the fridge to cool. After the curd has been inverted four times, remove the curd from the hoops and place into the cool water for 2 hours, 1 hour each side.

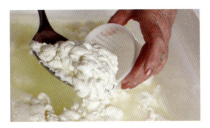

Next, make a brine solution by adding 200 g (7 oz) non-iodised salt into 1 litre (35 fl oz) of boiling water. Allow enough time for this to cool. Take the curd from the cold water and place into the brine solution for 3 hours, 1.5 hours on each side. Remove the curd from the brine solution and place onto a draining rack. Dry the cheese at room temp for 24 to 48 hours until dry.

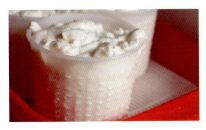

Day 2 or 3

When your cheese is feeling dry, it is ready to wax. Heat your cheese wax in an old but clean saucepan until it has just melted. Dip the cheese into the melted wax making sure it is well covered, usually about 3 layers is needed of wax to totally seal the cheese. Store you cheese at between 10–15°C (50–59°F) for 2 weeks, turning once a week. Your cheese is ready to eat at 2 weeks and can be stored in a regular fridge for up to 3 months.

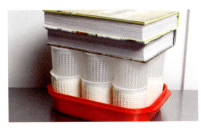

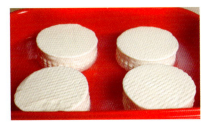

Affinage

The art of aging your cheese gracefully
In a lot of countries cheese is made on the farm or small factories, and then sent to the affineur to mature. It is their job to bring the cheese to its final ready state. In French, the word *affinage* simply means 'to refine', whether it is inoculating, washing, piercing and turning, making sure they are not too dry, not too wet, have enough air and not too much air. It really is an art, and it all depends on the style of the cheese.

What happens to the cheese in this maturing stage is loss of moisture, proteins breaking down, fats breaking down and the development of rinds, textures and flavors. Cheese is almost like a living thing and should be treated as such. Think of your maturing cheese as a low maintenance addition to the family, it needs a little looking after to encouraged it to age gracefully.

Being a home cheese maker means you have to be everything to your cheese, from start to finish. It really isn't that hard. I have been maturing cheese in a wine fridge successfully for the past 10 years. A wine fridge can be set at between 10°-15°C (50°-59°F), which is the perfect temperature to mature most of the cheeses you would be making at home. Wine fridges can be purchased from most stores that sell white goods. If you have a bar fridge that is not in use, electronic stores sell a thermostat that you can use as a replacement for the one in your bar fridge to increase the temperature. A tip with the bar fridge – unlike a wine fridge, a bar fridge has a fan which will dry your cheese out, so make sure you have your cheese in an air tight container to maintain the humidity, even place a little dish on water in the fridge. But remember your cheese needs air so don't forget to take it out of the fridge every day take the lid off and give it a turn, it will love you in return.

Waxing, vacuum sealing, and wrapping in cloth
Cheese is often aged with a coating to prevent air from contacting the surface of the cheese. When waxing or vacuum sealing a cheese not only will you be stopping air getting to the cheese you will be trapping anything that is inside the cheese in there as well. The cheese will also need to be totally air dry before waxing or vacuum sealing or it will weep.

Cloth wrapped cheese is just that, wrapping the cheese in cheese cloth. This is done after the final pressing, then air drying. Submerge the cloth in melted butter or lard I have used coconut oil as well, then wrap the cheese in the fatty cloth. Press the cheese again for approximately 12 hours. Remove the cheese from the press, wrap the cheese again in a second layer of cheese cloth and rub with oil. Press the cheese again for another 12 hours. The wrap should be smooth and snug; it's a bit like lining a cake tin, bottom, side and also a top. You may see some mould growing on the cloth and this can be removed by gently wiping with a mild brine solution. This method allows the cheese to breath but creates a barrier between it and the air.

Mould ripened cheeses

Some of the things to look out for when maturing a camembert is that the surface of the cheese needs the correct amount of moisture. How we achieve this is by creating a humid environment, do this be placing the lid onto the draining rack container. If the surface of the cheese is too moist the white mould which forms a rind over the cheese will not grow. This will leave the cheese exposed to the air for an extended period of time and the risk of bacterial contamination. If your allow the cheese to become too dry or allow it to dry too quickly, this will create a thick, white rind.

With blue cheeses, as with camembert and brie's, you need oxygen for the mould to grow. By piercing holes in your blue vein, this allows air pockets for the mould to grow and create veins.

Always remember that the best quality milk from grass fed cows and a clean environment are key factors in making high quality cheese. If these foundations are not in place, then your cheese will never be of a good quality. I always recommend supporting your local dairy farmer where possible and steering clearing of those "no name" brands.

Platter Suggestions

How do you go about creating the perfect cheese platter? With so many cheeses to choose from, creating the perfect pairing can be daunting. Think of mixing different textures, milk types and flavors on the one platter to keep things interesting. Do you want a light start to a meal? A decadent dessert platter? Work with the season, incorporate fruits that are in season, keep your lighter flavored cheeses for summer and your heavier/stronger flavors, like a washed rind, for winter.

Serving size 50–75 g (1¾–2½ oz) of cheese recommended per person.

Here are some of our favorites:

Platter 1 – Summer BBQ Antipasto Platter

A great way to showcase your homemade cheeses throughout the warm summer months.

Serve up a selection of baked ricottas, marinated fetta, Tzatziki from homemade yogurt and grilled haloumi. Serve with warm flatbread, olives, semidried tomatoes, marinated eggplant and watch it be devoured! Enjoy with a chilled glass of rose or cider.

Platter 2 – Autumn Dessert Platter

A dessert cheese plate is the perfect spread to serve after any meal. It's array of mouth-watering cheese combined with ginger, dark chocolate and nuts makes for a delicious alternative to a traditional dessert.

Dish up your homemade camembert, blue vein and cheddar with sides of biscotti, panforte, ginger snaps, glace figs, dark chocolate covered glaće ginger, glaće clementine's, nuts, plus grapes or other seasonal fruit.

Serve with a glass of your favorite dessert or fortified wine.

Platter 3 – Winter Entertaining Platter

The cooler months lead us to craving more complex, stronger and fuller flavors. This platter packs those bold flavors into one.

Start off with a warm, baked camembert, add washed rind, edam, cheddar and some of your stilton style blue vein. Serve with fresh bread, warm marinated olives, marmalade or relish. All you need is the bold red wine to top it off!

Platter 4 – Spring Platter

Now is the time to make the most of those beautiful fresh spring grasses and whip up some soft cheeses to really showcase the milk. Start off with some homemade boursin with fresh, in season herbs, add to your platter some chevre, a slice of double cream brie, creamy blue and monetary jack. Top it off with fresh strawberries, local honeycomb nuts and a fresh, crisp glass of white wine.

Your cheese is best served at room temperature, this allows the full flavors and aromas the develop. To prevent them from drying out cover with a clean damp tea towel.

Q & A

Why doesn't the Creamy Blue recipe have blue veins running through it?

The reason this happens is that the creamy blue is a soft cheese and although it is pierced to create an air pocket for the mould to grow, it often closes or collapses before the mould has a chance to grow through the vein. But don't despair, the flavor will be there without the mould, so let me explain further.

What creates the blue veining is the presence of Blue Mould Spore or Penicillium Roquefort which is introduced to the milk at the very beginning of the cheese making process. Now mould needs oxygen to grow, as a result, blue veins grow where the air pockets in the curd are. The size and dimension of these pockets are influenced by the curd's firmness. Cheese that become softer and creamier may display more, wispy veins, while curd with a firmer texture is less likely to collapse, maintaining the air pockets and giving a more shape and pattern to the veins. So next time you're making your creamy blue and you don't have any blue veins through the cheese, don't worry, it might look a little different but it will taste delicious even without them.

Why is my camembert too firm or runny?

Runny camembert is caused by not taking the temperature of the curd high enough in the cooking process. We cook the curd to give it the correct density for the white mould spore to work properly. as this grows on the outside to create the rind the white mould spore roots are working their magic to soften the cheese from the outside. Over cooking the curd will make the curd to dense and the cheese won't soften, under cooking the curd will make the curd not dense enough and the white mould spore will work quickly making a very soft cheese or if not cooked at all turning the inside back into a liquid.

Why won't my curd set after adding the rennet and mixing in?

Check these things; always dilute rennet in cool boiled water, boiling water removes the chlorine, chlorine will kill your rennet.

The milk used needs to be non-homogenised milk (not UHT).

The rennet is too old.

I don't have a clean break when checking the curd, it is still quite soft?

The temperature of the milk may have dropped, the lower the temperature of the milk the longer the set time. If the temperature has dropped to much you can pour some hot water into the styrene box to create a bay Marie to heat the milk up a little.

My yoghurt is too runny, what have I done?

Check these things:

Use UHT milk or heat fresh milk to 90°C (194°F) and cool to 40°C (104°F) before adding starter. Add 4 tablespoons of full cream milk powder. Leave in yoghurt maker for a minimum of 10 hours up to 16 hours.

Why am I getting less cheese from my milk than I did last time?

It could a seasonal thing. The richer the

pasture, the richer the milk, the more cheese or perhaps you have worked the curd more and released more whey.

Why is my cheese is bitter?
This can be caused by adding to much starter culture, rennet or mould spore. Other reasons are not enough whey has been removed, or there is to little salt added. Your equipment or work area is unclean, make sure everything is clean and sterile.

Why does my camembert smells like ammonia?
Your cheese needs to breathe, don't use cling wrap to wrap your cheese, wrap in baking paper and then foil works, or you can purchase cheese paper.

Why is my cheese like a sponge?
This is due to a contamination of culture perhaps with yeast or unwanted bacteria. Make sure you use high quality milk make sure your equipment is clean and sterile.

Can you freeze leftover cheese?
This is a question we get asked quite frequently and while we know a lot of people out there do freeze their cheeses, my recommendation is to please don't. Freezing of any cheese, both soft and hard cheeses, destroys the texture, which in turn affects the flavor, mouth feel and the enjoyment of eating cheese.

Do your best to enjoy your cheeses when they are ripe and ready for eating to get the full enjoyment from your homemade cheese, after all, that is what you make it for!

If you must freeze left over cheese, it is best then used for cooking as the texture is likely to be different to that your used to once it has thawed. In a recent experiment with freezing homemade Camembert, we found the flavor was ok (although not at its best), but the rind had started to fall off. Not exactly something you'd normally see on a cheese platter!

Cheeses are something to be shared and enjoyed, so if you find yourself with a whole lot of ready to eat cheeses, I'm sure you won't have any troubles finding someone to sit down with you to enjoy a glass of wine and a beautiful selection of your homemade cheese. That's what its all about.

Tricks of the trade

Now that you have read some of the recipes, how about changing some methods and/or ingredients to create your own new cheese? For a creamier cheese, try adding a little cream to the saucepan of milk when heating. Even 10ml of cream per litre can make a difference.

You can also adjust the moisture content of the cheese by cutting the curd either larger or smaller. The first cut of the curd is going to determine the amount of moisture that is in the cheese at the end of the day. The larger the cut the moister the cheese, the smaller the cut the drier the cheese. How this works is that the more cuts put into the curd the more whey is released, the less cuts the more whey is retained.

For added flavors in the cheese, why not try incorporating some dried herbs or spices to the curd before hooping. After you have removed as much whey as you can, stir through your chosen flavors. Easy, but very effective.

For a more pungent, stronger flavored cheese, leave in a humid environment for a little longer than the recipe suggests.

Sweeten yoghurts with icing sugar or runny honey. Anything that is heavier than the milk will just sink to the bottom of the pot. Don't forget - Never heat honey in the microwave! It kills all those good antioxidants and add your fruit when ready to eat.

If you are having trouble sourcing non-homogenised milk, you can create your own by using a 1 or 2% low fat milk and adding 40 ml (1½ fl oz) of pure cream per litre. So for 4 litres (135¼ fl oz) of low fat milk, add 160 ml (5½ fl oz) of pure cream when heating the milk. If using this methor it also helps to add a calcium solution at the same rate and at the same time as rennet in order to stabilise the milk.

Always remember to be hygienic and maintain a clean workspace.

Glossary

Aging is creating an environment to store the cheese at the correct temperature and humidity to develop the cheeses flavor, rind or consistency.

Bacteria or starter cultures are a lactic bacteria which start the fermentation process of cheese making. They replace the bacteria removed through pasturisation and give the cheese its flavor and character.

Blue mould spore is Penicillium roqueforti, it is added to the milk when making blue cheese.

Brevi Linens are used to create the sticky orange rind in washed rind cheese

Calcium solution is calcium chloride. It is added to low calcium milks such as goat's milk to help set a firmer curd. Or if you are using a homogenised milk and adding fresh cream to make your own non-homogenised milk.

Cheesecloth, not just a fabric that my wardrobe consisted of in the 70's. It is a finely woven material used to hang and/or wrap cheese so the whey can be released without losing any curd.

Cheese hoops give the cheese their final shape and assist in the draining of the whey from the curd.

Clean break this is to identifies the firmness of the curd, place the blade of a knife into the curd and lift at a 45-degree angle, looking for a clean break. If the curd parts well, it is ready to cut.

Cooking the curd the curd is heated to encourage more whey to be removed from the curd and changes the density of the curd.

Cutting the curd the curd is cut into equal size pieces, this is the first step for removing the whey. The more cuts that are put into the curd the more whey is removed and the firmer the cheese. The less cuts the more whey is retained the softer the cheese.

Curd & Whey after milk has been set and then cut, there is a solid white mass and a yellowish liquid. The mass is the curd and the liquid is the whey. Little miss Muffet suddenly makes sense!

Draining the whey is removing the whey prior to hooping the curd.

Drying or air drying the curd forms a rind prior to the aging process.

Enzymes always need to be diluted in boiled water, cooled. Lipase is used to break down fats and rennet to set curd.

Homogenisation is a process that disperses the fat molecules through the milk. This is done under extreme pressure, which changes the molecular structure of the milk. Rennet's job is to pull all the molecules in the milk together to set the curd. When using rennet use un or non homogenised milk.

Hooping the curd after the whey has been removed from the curd place it into the cheese hoops, the hoops give the cheese its shape.

Matuaration is creating an environment to store the cheese at the correct temperature and humidity to develop the cheeses flavor, rind or consistency.

Mould Spores Penicillin mould spores are used to create the rind, flavor, color and texture. The white mould spores used in the camembert recipe are penicillin candidum, blue cheese uses penicillin roquefort.

Pasteurization removes the natural accruing bacteria both good and bad that are in the milk.

Pressing the cheese removes whey, the more weight the more whey is removed.

Salt when making brine solutions or rubbing the surface of the cheese with salt you need to use non iodized salt, as iodine kills bacteria.

Starter cultures or bacteria are a lactic bacteria which start the fermentation process of cheese making. They replace the bacteria removed through pasteurization and give the cheese its flavor and character.

UHT milk is ultra heat treated, it is a long life milk sold on the supermarket shelf, it is convenient to use for quark, mascarpone and yoghurt as the milk needs to be sterile for the cultures to work. If using fresh milk to make these products you would need to heat the milk to 90°C (194°F) then cool.

Waxing applying a coat of cheese wax to the surface of the cheese to stop the cheese drying out and inhibit mould growth during the maturation or aging process.

Whey is the liquid that remains after the curd has been removed. We never through our whey away, our chooks drink the whey, I use the whey from the quark, mascarpone and labne in smoothies. Whey gets uses in our bread making or anywhere we use water in cooking.

Recipe Index

Creamy Blue	23
Stilton-Style Blue	25
Portobello Mushrooms with Blue Cheese & Sourdough Croutons	29
Potato Gnocchi with Blue Cheese Sauce	30
Bocconcini	33
Crumbed Bocconcini	34
Bocconcini Pin Wheels	37
Brie	39
Truffle Brie	43
Butter Cultured	45
Truffle Butter	46
Camembert	49
Camembert with Cranberries & Pistachios	53
Baked Camembert	53
Cheddar	55
Cheddar Washed Curd	58
Pull-apart Bread	61
Curds	63
Edam	65
Fetta	69
Persian Fetta	71
Spinach & Fetta Dip	73
Fetta Tart	74
Haloumi	77
Haloumi Hash with Eggs Benedict	81
Greek Baked Cheese	82
Havarti	85
Kefir	89
Mascarpone	91
Mascarpone & White Wine Fettuccine	92
Barrenjoey	95
Monterey Jack	97
Enchiladas	101
Jack & Beans	102

Mozzarella	105
Mozzarella & Basil Pizza	109
Paneer	111
Palak Paneer Curry	112
Quark	115
Homemade Boursin	117
Ricotta	119
Ricotta Gnocchi with Parmesan Broth	120
Ricotta Salata (poor man's parmesan)	123
Baked Ricotta Custard	124
Rag Pasta with Poor Man's Parmesan	127
Romano	129
Washed Rind	133
Fried Polenta and Mushrooms with Washed Rind	137
Greek Yoghurt	139
Labne	139
Tzatziki	140
Chèvre	143
Goat's Milk Fetta	144
Goat's Milk Havarti	146

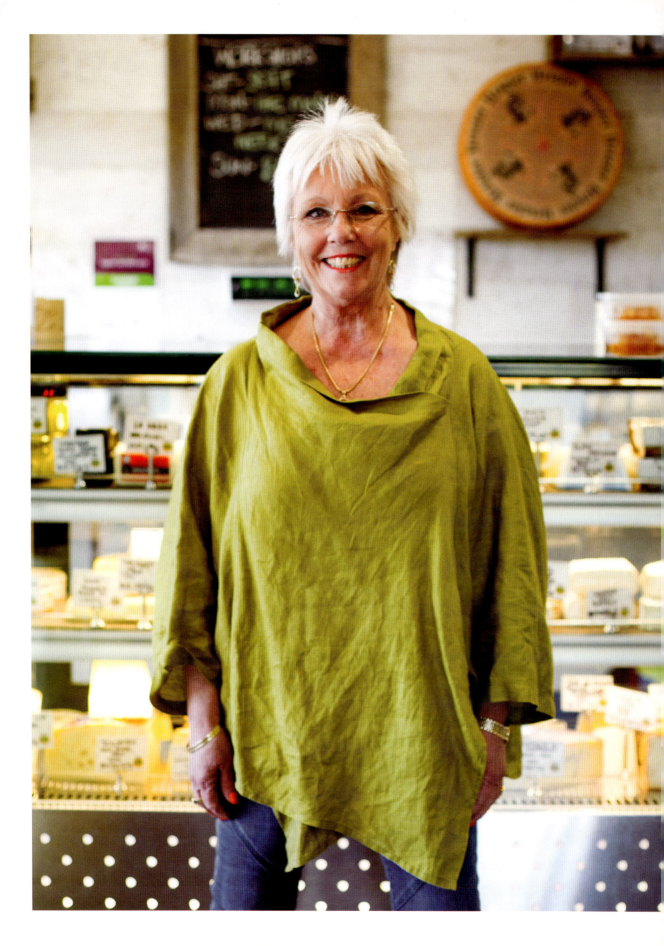

Acknowledgements

I would like to start by thanking my best friend Margie, who, through the ups and downs of business and life, has always been there for me. Her faith in my dream to spread the word of sustainability through cheesemaking has been unwavering. She has traveled far and wide with me on our road trips leaving her hubby John at home. We have had so much fun (AKA Thelma and Louise). I would like to thank my daughter Mel and our friend Ian for their patience in taking the photos of the cheesemaking process, making cheese is like watching paint dry. My hubby Wayne for being my rock and for his hard work and dedication. My daughter Mel who, since joining the business in 2015, has taken us on a massive journey, her words to me were "if your dreams don't scare you they aren't big enough". My son Wayne for being master cheese eater and recipe sampler. My sister Sue and her husband David for their support and assistance towards the growth of the business. And lastly, to those fellow cheese lovers that have attended our workshops.

About the author

Lyndall Dykes has been sharing her knowledge of cooking from scratch for more than three decades. After studying macrobiotics, she started a health food store in 1977, The Nut House. From there she taught vegetarian cooking classes in the region, before working in media, including sales and advertising on radio and Prime Television. At the same time Lyndall ran her family household where every staple item of food was made from scratch.

By 2006 she rekindled her passion for cheesemaking and in 2009 started teaching workshops from a purpose-built kitchen. She then created The Cheesemaking Workshop & Deli shopfront an the original plantation homestead. The only outlet of its kind in its country, the business is a one-stop haven for cheese devotees, and includes a deli – run by her daughter Melanie Browne – as well as teaching kitchens, dining room and equipment shop.

Lyndall and her workshops have been profiled on radio and in magazines and have featured extensively in regional and national news press. For years Lyndall regularly took her workshops on the road to assist those living in remote rural locations, as well as featuring at major food events.

In addition to being an award-winning businesswoman in her own right, Lyndall is a prominent voice among events and tourism industry bodies in her region. She sits on local government committees devoted to boosting food tourism for the region's local farmers, growers and restaurateurs.

To my very supportive family and friends and all the wonderful people I have met in my workshops.

A very special thank you to my daughter Mel who runs our very extensive cheese deli.

First published in 2018 by New Holland Publishers
London • Sydney • Auckland

131-151 Great Titchfield Street, London W1W 5BB, United Kingdom
1/66 Gibbes Street, Chatswood, NSW 2067, Australia
5/39 Woodside Ave, Northcote, Auckland 0627, New Zealand

newhollandpublishers.com

Copyright © 2018 New Holland Publishers
Copyright © 2018 in text: Lyndall Dykes
Copyright © 2018 in images: New Holland Publishers
Copyright © 2018 in step by step images: Lyndall Dykes

All rights reserved. No part of this publication may be reproduced, stored in a retrieval system or transmitted, in any form or by any means, electronic, mechanical, photocopying, recording or otherwise, without the prior written permission of the publishers and copyright holders.

A record of this book is held at the British Library and the National Library of Australia.

ISBN: 9781921024641

Group Managing Director: Fiona Schultz
Publisher: Monique Butterworth
Project Editor: Gordana Trifunovic
Proofreader: Kaitlyn Smith
Designer: Catherine Meachen
Photographer: Rebecca Elliot
Production Director: James Mills-Hicks
Printer: Toppan Leefung Printing Limited

10 9 8 7 6 5 4 3 2 1

OVEN GUIDE: You may find cooking times vary depending on the oven you are using. For fan-forced ovens, as a general rule, set the oven temperature to 20°C (35°F) lower than indicated in the recipe.

Keep up with New Holland Publishers on Facebook
www.facebook.com/NewHollandPublishers

UK 16.99
US 24.99